Summersdale Publishers Ltd
46 West Street
Chichester
West Sussex
PO19 1RP
UK

www.summersdale.com

Printed and bound by CPI Group (UK) Ltd, Croydon, CR0 4YY

ISBN: 978-1-84953-390-4

Substantial discounts on bulk quantities of Summersdale books are available to corporations, professional associations and other organisations. For details contact Nicky Douglas by telephone: +44 (0) 1243 756902, fax: +44 (0) 1243 786300 or email: nicky@summersdale.com.

Disclaimer
Every effort has been made to ensure that the information in this book is accurate and current at the time of publication. The author and the publisher cannot accept responsibility for any misuse or misunderstanding of any information contained herein, or any loss, damage or injury, be it health, financial or otherwise, suffered by any individual or group acting upon or relying on information contained herein. None of the opinions or suggestions in this book are intended to replace medical opinion. If you have concerns about your health, please seek professional advice.

Understanding and dealing with
Stroke

Foreword by Dr John Bamford MD FRCP
Consultant Stroke Physician and Stroke Association Trustee

Dr Keith Souter

PERSONAL HEALTH GUIDES ✚

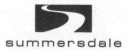

summersdale

For my sister-in-law, Mary

Acknowledgements

I would like to thank Isabel Atherton, my wonderful agent at Creative Authors for helping to bring this book to light. Thanks also to Claire Plimmer who commissioned the title and to my editor, Chris Turton, for the helpful suggestions and deft work with the editorial pen. Thanks also to Rachael Wilkie, my copy-editor, who helped to smooth out the manuscript. It has been a pleasure to work with them all.

Finally, a huge thank you to Dr John Bamford, an expert stroke physician and co-author of one of the major textbooks on stroke medicine, for taking the time out from his busy schedule to read the manuscript and write the foreword to the book.

Keith Souter

Contents

Venous thromboembolism
Dementia
Death

Foreword

By Dr John Bamford MD FRCP
Consultant Stroke Physician, Stroke Association Trustee

Strokes and transient ischaemic attacks can be frightening conditions for both stroke victims and their relatives. Whilst symptoms such as paralysis or loss of speech are well known consequences of stroke, it is often the myriad of more subtle changes to cognition and personality which cause as much, if not more, distress. It is natural to ask why these things happen, yet finding reliable and understandable explanations, even with all the power of the internet, can be extremely difficult. Furthermore, people want, and are able to assimilate, different levels of information at various points in their stroke journey.

The structure of this book by Keith Souter, a doctor and medical journalist, allows the reader to either dip in and out for specific pieces of information or read more deeply about the background to the problems. The style is both pragmatic and holistic, and he deals with the issues that we know are important to stroke victims and their carers but which often remain undiscussed. Understanding cannot repair the physical damage caused by a stroke but it can prevent or alleviate some of the emotional and psychological distress that is seen all too commonly. This book makes an extremely helpful contribution to that process.

'I'm not afraid of storms, for I'm learning how to sail my ship.'
Louisa May Alcott

Introduction

The term 'stroke' comes from antiquity, when medical knowledge was rudimentary. It was used to describe the way that someone in seemingly good health could suddenly develop loss of function of some part or parts of their body, or even suddenly die. It was assumed that they had been 'struck down' by God; hence, they had suffered a 'stroke'.

In fact, a stroke is the name that is given to a brain attack. In medicine, it used to be called a 'cerebrovascular accident'; however, this term is no longer considered adequate since no accident is involved. A stroke does not come about as the result of an injury from an accident, but is damage due to disruption of the blood supply to part of the brain, or from the rupture of a vessel to part of the brain.

Some can be fatal, some are totally disabling, others require varying lengths of time to recover from, and still others are purely temporary with a recovery time of less than twenty-four hours. The latter are called Transient Ischaemic Attacks (TIAs) or mini-strokes. Nonetheless, every single stroke (including a TIA) is a serious event and has to be dealt with as soon as possible to minimise and prevent further damage to the brain.

A stroke very often has a significant effect on other members of a family, since the person who has had the stroke may need considerable help with any resultant disabilities. It is often true to say that a stroke occurs in a moment, but can last a lifetime.

The aim of this book is to provide basic information to help readers understand strokes, so that they can deal with a stroke and its aftermath if they have one or if it happens to one of their family. It also gives information about how to spot risk factors that the reader or other members of their family should be aware of, in order to prevent a stroke or to reduce the risk of having a further one.

The book naturally falls into two parts. The first few chapters cover topics that you need to know about in order to understand how a stroke can produce various symptoms and different types of disability. The chapters in the second part cover topics that will help you to deal with a stroke and its repercussions.

Wherever appropriate, some basic facts and figures are given that you may find useful in terms of putting a stroke into the context of the topic under consideration. For example, Chapter 1 gives some statistics that will help you understand the way in which the brain is made up and how its size varies throughout life. In Chapter 2, there are statistics that tell you about the frequency of the different types of strokes.

Readers will vary in how much information they wish to absorb: some will want a full description and others will simply want the main points. In this book, I have tried to satisfy both types of reader. **Chapter 1, Understand the Brain**, contains a lot of information about this most complex of organs. I have indicated where the reader who wants to gloss over the bulk can go straight to the main facts; they may then decide whether they want to revisit the fuller description at a later stage. Also, to emphasise the main facts, boxes giving various key points appear throughout the book.

And so, to begin with, here are some general facts and figures about strokes:

- The World Health Organization estimated that in 2005 there were 5.7 million deaths from strokes worldwide.*

---

* www.who.int/chp/steps/stroke/en/index.html

- According to the World Stroke Organization, somewhere in the world someone dies from a stroke every six seconds and one person in six is liable to have a stroke in their lifetime.*

- In the UK, someone has a stroke every 5 minutes.

- There are approximately 110,000 first strokes in the UK per year.

- There are approximately 30,000 recurrent strokes in the UK per year.

- Strokes are the third most common cause of death (11 per cent of deaths in England and Wales).

- Strokes are the most common cause of long-term disability in the UK.

- There are 500,000 stroke victims living in the community in the UK.

  And also a few really key points:

- Strokes have nothing to do with heart attacks; a stroke is a 'brain attack'.

- Strokes are preventable.

- Strokes need emergency treatment, not a wait-and-see approach.

- Strokes can occur at any age; they are not restricted to the elderly.

- Stroke recovery continues for the rest of the person's life. It may be slow, but recovery is on-going.

---

* www.world-stroke.org

Part One

UNDERSTANDING STROKE

Your brain deserves respect

The human brain is an incredibly complex organ. However, like most of our internal parts, we tend to take it for granted until something goes wrong with it. The problem is that when something goes wrong, it can have catastrophic results. The brain is, after all, the control centre of the body, the computer that governs the way that most of the body functions; it processes all of the incoming information and it calculates what you need to do about it.

A stroke can suddenly disrupt many of these vital functions. It can be a confusing event, because often it occurs without any warning, without any pain and, it may seem, without any mercy.

In this first part of the book we look at the brain and try to give an understanding about the way that it works. We then look at the different types of stroke in order to see just how a stroke can produce the sort of symptoms and problems that it does. By understanding the pathology you will be better able to understand the aims of treatment and rehabilitation when we come to look at them in Part 2.

Chapter 1

Understand the brain

The brain is the most important organ in the body; it controls movement and is the organ which perceives all of the information that is transmitted from the sense organs through touch, vision, hearing, smell and taste. It is also where you perceive pain. You might say that the brain is the essence of the individual, since it is where all of our thought processes and emotions seem to take place; that is, the brain seems to be the seat of the mind. This is a very interesting point, which has been widely debated by philosophers and scientists almost since the beginning of human consciousness. We will come back to this later in the chapter, since it is important in our understanding of the brain.

Figure 1

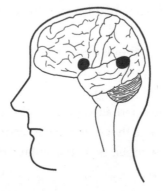

Basic brain facts

- The average adult brain weighs about 3 lb.

- The brain has a texture like firm jelly.

- The brain is made up about one hundred billion cells.

- About a quarter of the blood pumped out by the heart with every heartbeat goes to supply the brain.

- The brain uses about 20 per cent of the body's oxygen.

- The brain needs a continuous supply of oxygen. A few minutes of oxygen deprivation will lead to irreversible damage.

- The brain looks wrinkled and not unlike a walnut. Those wrinkles are called convolutions and they are where you do your thinking.

The nervous system

The nervous system is the body's main communication system. It is customary to consider it as having two parts – the central nervous system, consisting of the brain and spinal cord, and the peripheral nervous system, consisting of the nerves to the various parts of the body.

The nervous system controls every aspect of your bodily function, ranging from the involuntary processes like breathing to the voluntary processes of moving. The brain, of course, is the great computer of the body where all the information from sensory nerves is transmitted and where thoughts and decisions are made, and it is from there that nerve impulses are transmitted down motor nerves to make muscles move.

This next section considers the brain in a little more depth and shows how we have come to build up a picture of the brain. If you simply want to quickly get an idea of the basic structure of the brain then you can skip ahead to **The basic brain structures in medicine** on page 34. You can of course return later if you want to gain a deeper understanding.

What the ancients thought about the brain

We know that our early ancestors recognised that the head was often the site of illness. In a time when the world and the universe seemed to be under the control of gods, people understandably thought that illness and disease resulted when the gods were angry or when spirits possessed an individual.

Archaeological evidence shows that the practice of trephination, the boring of a hole in the skull, was used in early tribal societies. It was presumably thought that this would let out evil spirits. Examination of many skulls which had been trepanned in this way shows that healing of bone around the site of the boring often took place, indicating that in many cases the operation was a success. Incredibly, they used three distinct methods – cutting, scraping and drilling.

The reason that the procedure could have helped some people with head injuries or certain other conditions was because it would have released pressure upon the brain; a head injury could have caused a rise in pressure, resulting in bleeding inside the skull. Unfortunately, for those people who were not suffering from a rise in pressure, the trephination may have done actual harm.

The ancient Egyptians had developed a quite sophisticated system of medicine and surgery with doctors who specialised in one area of the body. Thus, they had eye doctors, stomach doctors and head surgeons. The Edwin Smith Papyrus, written in about 1500 BC, is essentially an Egyptian textbook of surgery. It describes surgical instruments and techniques and discusses 48 cases of injuries, including head injuries.

A beautiful description of ancient Egyptian surgery is given in the 1945 historical novel *The Egyptian* by the Finnish writer, Mika Waltari, which became an international bestseller, and later a Hollywood blockbuster in 1954. In the novel, the main character, Sinuhe, who would become the royal physician to Pharaoh Akhenaten, is apprenticed to Ptahor, the 'opener of heads'. Ptahor shows him how to examine a patient and diagnose where there may be a problem in the head from an assessment of the state of consciousness and the use of the limbs. He then shows him how to remove a piece of skull and replace it with a silver plate which is bound with bandages while the patient awaits recovery.

The Greeks abhorred the thought of anatomical dissection, so most of their theories about brain function came through simple observation. The great philosopher and scientist, Aristotle, incorrectly taught that the heart was actually the organ that controlled thought and emotions. He described the way that people with heavy upper bodies were often slow witted, as a result of the drain on their heart.

In about 450 BC, the ancient Greek physician, Hippocrates, known as the father of medicine, described the condition of stroke. He called it apoplexy, which literally meant 'struck down by violence'. This archaic term was used right up until the twentieth century.

The rise of anatomy

In the second century the Greek physician Claudius Galenus of Pergamum (AD 131–201), better known as Galen, performed several dissections on animals and accurately described many of the organs of the body. He described the function of the nerves, and examined the structures of the eyes, ears, larynx and the reproductive organs. He taught that psychic gases and humours flowed through the body into the ventricles of the brain, thereby allowing the development of mental functions.

After that, the Church banned the anatomical dissection of the body and it was not until the sixteenth century that further advances in knowledge about the brain were made. Andreas Vesalius (1514–1564) was a Flemish anatomist who demonstrated that Galen and other early anatomists had been incorrect in some of their conclusions. In 1543, he wrote the first anatomically accurate medical textbook, *De Humani Corporis Fabrica* (*On the Fabric of the Human Body*), which was complete with precise illustrations.

One of King Charles II's physicians was Dr Thomas Willis (1621–1675). He was an anatomist who was deeply interested in the blood supply of the body. He published several books in the 1660s, the most significant being a work about the brain. In it, he described the circle of blood vessels at the base of the brain, which was formed from major arteries travelling up the front of the neck and joining with ones from the back of the neck, to produce an arterial circle which gave off branches to supply blood to the various areas of the brain. This is called the Circle of Willis. We shall look at it in more detail in the next chapter.

Contemporary with Willis was Johan Jacob Wefner (1620–1695), a Swiss physician who discovered that some patients who died from apoplexy had actually had a bleed into the brain. He also concluded that blockage of one of the main blood vessels in the brain could produce apoplexy. In 1658, he published a great treatise, *Historiae apoplecticorum*, or *History of Stroke*. It is one of the classic texts on strokes.

The nineteenth century – major advances

The Victorian era saw an explosion in knowledge in all areas of science, medicine included. It was not always a straightforward progression of knowledge, however, as was shown by the development of a pseudo-science called phrenology. This was an idea introduced by an Austrian physician called Franz Gall, who suggested that the brain consisted of a collection of individual faculties, each of which was associated with a different mental function, character quality or emotion. Phrenologists 'read' the lumps and bumps on people's heads in order to read their characters. You can still see phrenological busts and maps of the head with all of these 'faculties' outlined and numbered in a network over the head in various textbooks of psychology. The theory has died out, yet the iconic image lives on.

Yet this misconception that specific functions could be localised was taken up by many doctors and led to further misconceptions about the brain and the mind. Gradually, it became clearer that, while there were some parts of the brain that seemed to have specific roles, by and large the brain worked as a single organ – so that if damage or injury occurred in one part, other parts could eventually take over that function.

There are three major discoveries that we should consider:

The speech centre

In the mid-nineteenth century, the French surgeon and anthropologist Pierre-Paul Broca (1824–1880) discovered that the left hemisphere of the brain was dominant in speech production. He localised this to a very specific area in the frontal lobe of the dominant hemisphere. It was named after him as Broca's area.

Language comprehension

Not long after Broca's discovery, Carl Wernicke (1848–1905), a German anatomist and psychiatrist, discovered another area of the brain associated with the way that we understand language and writing. This was also found in the dominant hemisphere, but is towards the back of the temporal area: it is known as Wernicke's area.

Memory

The Russian psychiatrist Sergei Korsakoff (1854–1900) studied the effects of alcoholism. He found that in advanced cases patients became paranoid, developed memory problems and could eventually manifest a type of movement disorder or stagger that is called ataxia. From anatomical examination of the brains of people with such problems he found that they had developed a specific nutritional deficiency (later found to be vitamin B1 or thiamine), which caused structural changes in areas of the middle of the brain. He deduced that these areas were associated with the ability to remember. As a result, we now know that the temporal lobes of the brain are associated with memory function.

The parts of the brain

We are now in a position to have a look at the different parts of the brain, in order to see what parts control which aspects of our body functions.

> **Please note** that in this section we are going to discuss the brain in a logical manner from a biological sense, to give you an understanding of how the brain works functionally. Later, in the section on the basic parts of the brain, we consider the parts in a slightly different way, as we do in medicine. This will be helpful in distinguishing how different types of stroke cause different clinical patterns of symptoms.

The evolved brain Human beings are the most evolved creatures on the planet in terms of brain function. Our brains are similar to other primates, all of which are more evolved than other mammals. In turn, all mammalian brains are more evolved than the brains of birds or reptiles.

When we look at the brain in this sense we can see how our brains have evolved, for we have three parts that reflect the advance up the evolutionary tree.

Brain comparisons

If you scale mammals, birds and reptiles to the same body size, the mammal would have a brain twice as large as a bird and ten times as large as a reptile's. A mammalian brain is twice as large as a bird's brain.

Here we need to look inside the brain, so take a look at Figure 2 which shows a section through the brain from front to back. This shows the three main parts of the brain. They reflect the development of the brain up the evolutionary tree.

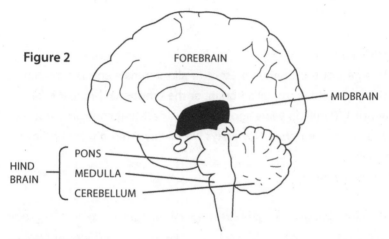

Figure 2 FOREBRAIN

MIDBRAIN

HIND BRAIN { PONS
MEDULLA
CEREBELLUM

The hindbrain

This part of the brain is sometimes called the 'reptilian brain', because it is present in reptiles. It evolved hundreds of millions of years ago. It is the part of the brain that takes care of our basic life functions, such as control of our heartbeat, our breathing. It is also our instinctive brain which controls our survival need, our sexual desires and our basic needs.

It consists of:

- The spinal cord – which relays information to and from the brain to the rest of the body.

- The medulla oblongata – which controls all the autonomic functions. These are the involuntary functions of the body like the heartbeat, breathing and digestion.

- The pons – which regulates sleep and controls one's level of consciousness.

- The cerebellum – the large structure at the back and the bottom of the brain, which controls movement and balance. It has a right and a left hemisphere.

The midbrain

This part of the brain is present in all mammals and is sometimes called the 'old mammalian brain', or the 'emotional brain'. It evolved about 150 million years ago. This is the part that controls emotions and stores memories. Nowadays we mainly refer to it as the 'limbic system'.

It consists of:

- The amygdala – an almond-shaped structure (its name being the Latin for 'almond'), which has a role in storing deep emotional memories. It seems to control fear and is responsible for activating all the unpleasant sensations we experience when frightened, such as palpitations, butterflies in the stomach, sweaty hands and shivers. There is also mounting evidence that it is associated with addictive tendencies.

- The hippocampus – which is involved in memory-storing and memory-processing. It is shaped a little like a seahorse, hence its name, which comes from the Greek.

- The hypothalamus – is the workhorse of the brain, in terms of regulating many of our internal functions, such as thirst, appetite, internal balance of metabolism, temperature control and circadian rhythms such as the sleep cycle.

- The thalamus – which is the great signal box of the brain. It relays information from all of the sense organs to the higher parts of the brain where the information is processed and the experiences of the senses are perceived. It has a large part to play in pain perception as well as being the relay centre for movements.

The forebrain

The forebrain is also called the neocortex, or the neomammalian brain, or the 'rational brain'. It is the last part of the brain to have evolved and is found in other primates as well as in highly intelligent mammals like dolphins.

It makes up two thirds of the whole brain and it is where we think, perceive, create and plan. It is where we organise thoughts to produce language, solve problems, philosophise and experience life.

It is also where we perceive all the information from our sense organs and control our body movements.

The hemispheres

There are two halves of the neocortex, called hemispheres. Certain functions of the mind seem to be associated with either the right and left hemispheres of the brain. This has become known as the 'right brain v. left brain' theory of mind. It was based on the work of psycho-biologist Robert Sperry (1913–1994), for which he received a Nobel Prize in 1981.

Sperry's work gave us some very good insight into the brain–mind connection and delineated functions that seem more associated with one hemisphere than the other. It does not mean that they are exclusively associated in that way, for other work indicates that, in many ways, the brain is holographic. This means that all parts of the brain have the potential to operate the mind, so that if there is injury to one part of the organ other parts may be able to take over function. So it is more an order of pre-eminence of associations rather than exclusive association.

Table 1 Right and left hemisphere associations

RIGHT HEMISPHERE	LEFT HEMISPHERE
Visual	Verbal
Intuitive	Logical
Creative	Analytical
Artistic	Scientific
Musical	Mathematical
Lateral thinking	Linear thinking
Emotions	Clinical
Physically expressive	Verbally expressive
Hears nuances	Hears sounds
Poor time sense or awareness	Good time sense and awareness
Poor organisation	Good organisation
Pattern recognition – sees pictures	Item recognition – sees links

Its significance is that some people seem to be more one-sided than the other; in other words, the operation of their brains and minds seems to be biased towards one hemisphere. Thus, we talk about right-hemisphere dominance or left-hemisphere dominance. Once again, it is important to appreciate that this does not mean that only one side works, but that the functions of one side seem to be most to the fore in the way that these people think and live.

The two hemispheres are connected by a part of the brain called the corpus callosum. This is a bridge where nerve pathways pass over from one hemisphere to the other side of the body. This results in the left side of the brain controlling the right side of the body, and the right hemisphere controlling the left side of the body.

The lobes

Each hemisphere of the neocortex has four lobes, each of which has a different function (see Figures 3(a) and 3(b)).

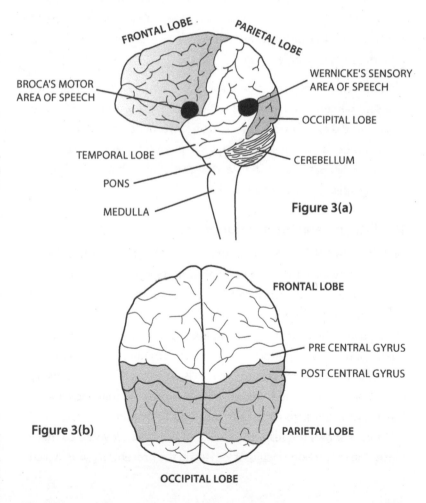

Figure 3(a)

Figure 3(b)

- The frontal lobe – where reasoning, calculation, problem solving and judgement take place. Broca's area is usually in the frontal lobe.

- The parietal lobe – where pain and touch are processed.

- The temporal lobe – which is mainly concerned with memory, although it is also associated with emotions and speech. Wernicke's area, which controls language recognition, is located in the temporal lobe in the left hemisphere. Sound is also perceived in the temporal lobes.

- The occipital lobe – at the back of the brain, is associated with visual perception. This may be the most surprising finding, since one would expect visual perception to occur near to the eyes, but in fact quite complex pathways are involved. We shall consider these when we come to the section on visual problems in **Chapter 8, Complications after a stroke.**

The little person inside your brain

Dr Wilder Penfield (1891–1976), an American neurosurgeon, did a lot of research work in the mid-twentieth century while treating patients with epilepsy, which advanced our understanding of the way the brain perceives the body.

Effectively, there are two maps spread out across parts of the brain: one is for organising motor function, which operates our movements; the other is a sensory map, which is where all of the sensory information is processed. Wilder Penfield suggested that each map is like a homunculus, from the Latin meaning 'little man'.

Figure 4 shows the respective areas of the brain devoted to these maps. The motor homunculus is located in the precentral gyrus, which is the back edge of the frontal lobe. The sensory homunculus is located in the postcentral gyrus, which is the front edge of the parietal lobe.

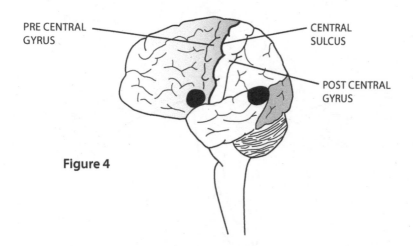

PRE CENTRAL
GYRUS

CENTRAL
SULCUS

POST CENTRAL
GYRUS

Figure 4

If you now look at Figure 5(a), showing the brain in profile through the postcentral gyrus, you will see the relative areas of the brain that are devoted to sensation, giving an impression of how the brain 'sees' the body. It is effectively like an upside-down, small person with big feet, huge hands, a large head with prominent eyes, ears, nose and big tongue (see figure 5(b)).

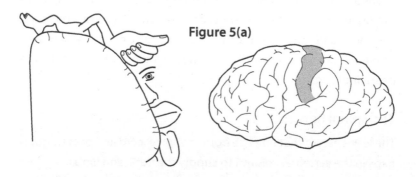

Figure 5(a)

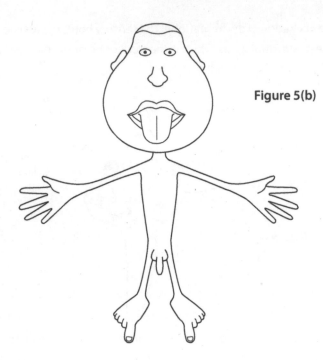

Figure 5(b)

And if you think about it, that is what it feels like, although our brains give us a more aesthetic perception of ourselves.

The cranial nerves

There are twelve pairs of special nerves that emerge directly from the brain. Some of these carry sensory information from the eyes, ears, nose and mouth, and others control muscles of the head and throat. Yet others supply various glands or important organs like the heart and lungs.

The spinal nerves

These are nerves that emerge from the spinal cord and pass through gaps in the vertebral column to supply the trunk and limbs.

To summarise:

- The human brain is the most evolved of all the mammalian brains. Viewed from an evolutionary basis, there are three brains in one – the hindbrain, midbrain and forebrain.

- The left side of the brain controls the movements of the right side of the body, and the right side of the brain controls the left side of the body.

- The spinal cord runs down inside the vertebral column or spine, giving off spinal nerves to supply the various parts of the body.

- Cranial nerves come off directly from the brain to supply the head and neck and various internal organs like the heart and lungs.

The mind and the brain

Most people feel that their personality, their consciousness – indeed, all those things that give an individual a sense of self – are located inside their head. It is as if the individual is inside the head, looking out at the world beyond.

As we saw earlier, Aristotle thought that the heart, rather than the brain, was the seat of the emotions. The reason for this probably related to the observation that the heart speeds up whenever someone gets excited or when they are anxious. From what we have already discussed throughout this chapter it is clear that mind processes take place inside the brain.

Psychologists and neurobiologists are nowadays fortunate in having two very effective types of scanners called functional Magnetic Resonance Imaging (fMRI) and Positive Emission

Tomography (PET). These are allowing researchers to virtually picture what is happening inside the brain during certain activities or when someone is thinking different types of thought.

Although it is something of an oversimplification, we can basically say that the functions of the mind mirror the anatomy of the brain that we have so far considered:

- The rational mind is associated with the functioning of the frontal lobes.

- Creativity and artistic ability seem to be right-hemisphere functions of mind.

- Logic and mathematical ability seem to be left-hemisphere functions of the mind.

- Our emotional mind seems to be associated with the limbic system or the midbrain.

- Our instinctive mind processes seem to be associated with the brainstem.

The brainstem

In medicine, it is common to consider the midbrain and the pons and medulla as the brainstem. This is because doctors can clinically make a diagnosis and evaluation of how well a patient may recover from a particular kind of stroke.

The whole question about the nature of the mind is not cut and dried. There is huge debate in scientific, philosophical and religious circles about whether it is something that is separate from brain function, or simply a sort of by-product of brain function, rather like the noise that is produced by a machine.

The French philosopher René Descartes (1596–1650) believed that mind and body were definitely separate and that only humans had been blessed with a thinking mind. His famous utterance, *cogito, ergo sum*, meaning 'I think, therefore I am', is the essence of the so-called Cartesian dualism that dominated Western philosophy for centuries.

Against this, many neuroscientists suggest that the mind is generated by brain activity. It is beyond our remit to say what the mind is, but it seems clear that brain activity and mental and emotional functions are linked. The effects of drugs and alcohol, for example, affect brain function and, as a result, thoughts and emotions may be affected. This also helps us to understand how damage to part or parts of the brain from stroke can affect mental processes and emotions.

Thinking and non-thinking parts of the nervous system – grey matter and white matter

If you enjoy the crime fiction of Agatha Christie then you may well have read of her detective, Hercule Poirot, saying that 'it is a case for the little grey cells'. He refers to the thinking part of the brain, the grey cells that compose the grey matter.

The outer part or the surface of the brain gets its colour from the type of nerve cells that it contains – these are the bodies of the nerve cells; they have no covering of myelin, hence their grey-pink appearance.

The cerebral cortex and most of the cerebellum consists of grey matter, as does the central core of the spinal cord.

The deeper tissue of the brain and cerebellum and the outer part of the spinal cord and the peripheral nerves are made up of myelinated nerve fibres. These make up the white matter. Essentially, this is the conducting tissue, or the 'wiring' part of the system.

In summary, the thinking parts of the brain are made of grey matter and the non-thinking, wiring parts, consist of white matter.

The basic brain structures in medicine

I said earlier that the description of the brain in a biological sense helps us to understand how it has evolved over millions of years. It is essentially three ever more complex developments, or three brains in one.

In the context of understanding how the brain controls the body, in medicine we consider it in a slightly different manner. What follows is therefore the information that you need to be aware of in order to understand how a stroke can affect the individual.

The nervous system consists of the brain and spinal cord and the peripheral nerves. Working together, they control every part of your body, both the involuntary and important aspects such as breathing and the rate of the heart, and the voluntary processes such as moving muscles and walking.

The brain has three main parts, as we discussed in the section on the evolving brain. These are the forebrain, the midbrain and the hindbrain. In medicine, it is usual to consider the midbrain, pons and medulla all together as the brainstem.

Thus in medicine we label the following regions as the three parts of the brain:

1. The cerebrum, consisting of the two cerebral hemispheres.

2. The cerebellum, consisting of two cerebellar hemispheres.

3. The brainstem.

The cerebrum
This makes up two-thirds of the whole brain and it is where we think, perceive, create and plan. It is where we organise thoughts to produce language, solve problems, philosophise and experience life.

It is also where we perceive all the information from our sense organs and control our body movements.

The cerebrum is made up of a right hemisphere and a left hemisphere. The right hemisphere controls the left side of the body and the left hemisphere controls the right side of the body.

Each cerebral hemisphere has four lobes (see Figure 3):

- The frontal lobe – where reasoning, calculation, problem solving and judgement take place. Broca's area, which controls speech, is usually in the frontal lobe.

- The parietal lobe – where pain and touch are processed.

- The temporal lobe – which is mainly concerned with memory, although it is also associated with emotions and speech. Wernicke's area, which controls language recognition, is located in the temporal lobe in the left hemisphere. Sound is also perceived in the temporal lobes.

- The occipital lobe – at the back of the brain, is associated with visual perception. This may be the most surprising finding, since one would expect visual perception to occur near to the eyes, but in fact quite complex pathways are involved. We shall consider these when we come to the section on visual problems in **Chapter 8, Complications after a stroke**.

Most people have a dominant hemisphere. In the majority of right-handed people the left hemisphere is dominant. This tends to be the hemisphere which contains the speech centres, so if a right-handed person has a left-hemisphere stroke they will experience speech problems and will have right side of body paralysis and sensory loss.

You would imagine that, similarly, the majority of naturally left-handed people would have a dominant right hemisphere. This is not always the case. About 50 per cent have dominance of the right and 50 per cent have dominance of the left hemisphere.

The cerebellum

The cerebellum is the large structure at the back and the bottom of the brain, which controls the coordination of movement and balance. It has a right and a left hemisphere, like a miniature cerebrum.

The brainstem

This is the part of the brain that is made up of the midbrain, pons and medulla. It basically controls all of the vital life functions, such as heartbeat, blood pressure and breathing.

This completes our little journey through the nervous system. We now know enough about the different parts of the brain to understand why a stroke produces some of its symptoms.

Chapter 2

What happens in a stroke

A stroke is always a serious event

A stroke is the name given to a 'brain attack' in which an area of the brain is deprived of its blood supply. The blood supplies the brain with oxygen and nutrients, including glucose. If the blood supply is cut off to a part of the brain then the delicate brain cells will start to become damaged and quickly die off. This takes place within a mere six minutes, so time is of the essence.

It is important to appreciate that a stroke is always a serious event and should be treated as a medical emergency. Permanent damage to the brain can occur, or even death.

During a stroke the blood supply can be affected in two main ways:

1. Ischaemia

This means that a blockage occurs in a blood vessel. Generally, this is the result of cholesterol plaques building up inside the vessel. Essentially, it is a result of hardening of the arteries.

There are two ways that an ischaemic stroke occurs. One way is if a plaque on a brain blood vessel ruptures then a clot rapidly forms about the damaged area. If this is large enough to block the flow of blood then the part of the brain supplied by that blood vessel may be damaged.

The other way is if a clot forms in another part of the body and flows along the circulation to lodge in a narrow part of an artery supplying the brain. This also produces ischaemia. Such a clot is called an embolus.

2. Haemorrhage

This is when a blood vessel bursts, and bleeds into the brain itself.

How circulation works

William Harvey (1578–1657) was a physician and anatomist who fought in the English Civil War and who was court physician to three kings of England. After much research on animals he demonstrated the circulation of the blood and announced his discovery of the circulatory system in 1616. In 1628, he published his work *Exercitatio Anatomica de Motu Cordis et Sanguinis in Animalibus* (*An Anatomical Exercise on the Motion of the Heart and Blood in Animals*). It was arguably the most significant piece of medical research ever written and laid the foundation for the scientific study of medicine. He proposed that blood flowed through the heart in two separate loops, a pulmonary circulation going to the lungs and another, the systemic circulation, going to the organs, including the brain and the extremities.

Key points about circulation

Effectively, the heart is like two pumps joined together. The left side of the heart receives oxygenated (oxygen-rich) blood from the lungs and pumps it out to the organs and tissues. This is called the systemic circulation, and the brain receives its supply of blood from the systemic circulation. The right side of the heart receives deoxygenated (oxygen-depleted) blood from the tissues and pumps it out to the lungs to collect more oxygen. This is called the pulmonary circulation.

Arteries carry blood away from the heart to the organs and tissues, and veins carry it back to the heart.

Arteries carry oxygenated blood to the tissues to nourish them. Veins carry deoxygenated blood back to the heart, in order to be pumped to the lungs to receive more oxygen.

Capillaries are tiny, thread-like blood vessels that join the arterial circulation to the venous circulation. They feed the tissues.

The blood supply to the brain

The brain is the most important organ in the body, It is made up about one hundred billion cells, all of which have to receive a continuous supply of oxygen from the blood. The circulation of blood to the brain is therefore crucial to our understanding of strokes, since it is deprivation of oxygen to a part of the brain that results in a stroke.

As mentioned in Chapter 1, the blood supply to the brain was discovered by Dr Thomas Willis in the mid-seventeenth century (see Figure 6). Essentially, the two internal carotid arteries in the front of the neck pass up into the skull and form a ring with vessels from the basilar artery, which is itself formed from two vertebral arteries which pass up the back of the neck into the back of the skull. This ring is called the Circle of Willis and is located underneath the brain.

Smaller arteries then branch off from it and travel upwards to supply very specific parts of the brain.

When someone has a stroke it may be possible on the basis of the clinical examination to deduce which part of the brain has been affected. Further investigation, including various types of scan, may pinpoint the site of the lesion and determine the nature of the damage.

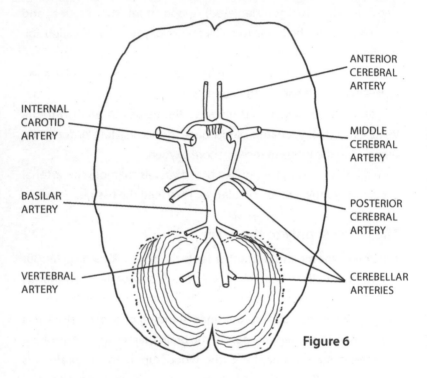

Figure 6

Thus, the following branches supply:

- Anterior cerebral arteries – supply the front of the brain and the motor and sensory areas for the lower part of the body. A blocked anterior cerebral artery may cause paralysis and sensory deficit on the opposite side of the body from the hips down. There can also be incontinence of the bowel or the bladder. Since it also supplies the frontal area, some personality change can occur.

- Middle cerebral arteries – supply the areas involved in speech, swallowing and language function. The middle cerebral arteries supply a large part of the brain, including the corpus striatum. This is involved in regulating our movements, and so can result in a wide variety of problems. A stroke affecting the middle cerebral artery can also cause a specific visual defect called hemianopsia, which can result in the loss of half of the visual field in each eye. We shall look at and explain this in **Chapter 8, Complications after a stroke**.

- Posterior cerebral arteries – supply a lot of the hind part of the brain. Since this area has a large part to play in vision, a wide variety of visual problems can be associated with a stroke affecting this area.

- Cerebellar arteries – supply the cerebellum, so they are often associated with ataxia or balance and coordination problems.

KEY POINTS

The Circle of Willis can actually protect you from having a stroke. The fact that there is a circle means that if one vessel becomes blocked, then the blood can still find its way to the area of the brain by means of some of the other vessels. It varies from person to person. Some people may block one vessel and suffer a stroke while other people can block two or more vessels and yet have no symptoms.

The fact is that anatomy varies from one person to another. Some have a well-formed circle and therefore may have a good collateral circulation (meaning circulation to a part of the brain by several vessels), whereas in some people it is not fully formed. In the former case they may be able to sustain a clot on one part but be able to maintain a circulation to prevent brain cell death. In the latter, with a less developed Circle of Willis, a blockage could be catastrophic.

Blockage or bleed – the different causes of a stroke

Broadly there are two main causes of strokes – ischaemic ones (blockages) and haemorrhagic ones (bleeds).

Ischaemic strokes

Ischaemic strokes account for about 80 per cent of strokes.

'Ischaemia' means being deprived of blood; this can come about through narrowing of an artery, a thrombosis or clot, or from the impact of an embolus, a clot that has been carried from elsewhere in the body to lodge in and block a brain vessel.

Hardening of the arteries

The medical term for the problem that underlies a lot of ischaemic strokes is arteriosclerosis. It is commonly referred to as hardening of the arteries.

Blood vessels have a lining of a single layer of epithelial cells. As long as this epithelial lining is intact, then the blood flows smoothly.

If you think of arteries as being like rivers, then you can get an idea of the way arteriosclerosis will build up. It is a bit like silting up of a river. At bends in the blood vessels, there will be a tendency for silting to take place. It does not just result in a deposit like sand, but in the build-up of what's called atheroma plaque.

The plaque is rather like a fatty streak in a vessel wall. Fat molecules get absorbed through the epithelial lining to form a swelling in the vessel wall. Calcium and other minerals may also get trapped in it and fibrous tissue forms to create a hard lumpiness that will narrow the calibre of the vessel and also make it harder and less flexible.

Lots of plaques can develop along the course of an artery, the net effect being to narrow it along a significant length, thereby reducing the flow of blood through it. If this happens in the coronary arteries which supply the heart, then angina may be the result. If it happens in the circulation to the brain, then it can start to produce cerebral ischaemia. This means that the brain is being deprived of oxygen. These gradually narrowing vessels become more likely to get blocked by a blood clot.

Thrombosis

As long as the integrity of the epithelial lining is maintained, then the blood will flow. However, if that layer is disrupted by the rupture of a plaque, then messenger chemicals will alert blood cells which will move to the area to form a clot to seal off the damaged part of the vessel. Platelets will accumulate and a fibrous structure like a spider's web will be formed to catch more cells to help to seal the damage. This is called a thrombus.

The process of thrombus formation is called thrombosis.

If a cerebral artery is very narrow and the thrombus becomes big enough to block off the flow of blood, then a brain attack or stroke occurs.

An ischaemic stroke can be of these three varieties:

- Transient Ischaemic Attack (TIA) – this is a brain attack that lasts less than 24 hours. The blockage is only transient and normal flow is re-established by the body. It must be treated seriously, however, since it may be a warning of a serious major stroke.

- Cerebral thrombosis – this is the formation of a blood clot in one of the cerebral arteries that is already narrowed and partially furred up.

- Cerebral embolism – here, a clot that has arisen in another part of the body is hurled into the cerebral circulation and lodges in a narrowed artery. The likeliest cause is an irregular heartbeat, such as atrial fibrillation, but clots are also possible in the following conditions:

  - Atrial fibrillation
  - Auto-immune disorders
  - Bleeding disorders like hemophilia
  - Certain cancers
  - Genetic factors, e.g. CADASIL (see Chapter 4)
  - Heart failure
  - Heart valve disease
  - High blood pressure
  - Severe infection
  - Trauma to a blood vessel due to a recent heart attack or stroke.

Lacunar stroke

So far we have considered strokes that occur when one of the main arteries or a main branch from the Circle of Willis is affected. There are many much smaller blood vessels that branch off from these larger arteries; these extend deep into the substance of the brain. When these smaller blood vessels get blocked, a lacunar stroke may be the result. This tends to occur in long-standing conditions, such as atherosclerosis in old age, diabetes and hypertension, which have caused previous narrowing of the blood vessel. When a clot forms in one of these small, deep vessels it will cause a lacunar stroke.

The term is used because the brain typically shows a lacuna, which is Latin for 'empty space'. It can take years for this space to form after the original stroke. It occurs because when one of these little blood vessels is blocked, it is like blocking a cul-de-sac, so that the small area beyond the block eventually just melts away to become a space, like the hole in a sponge.

Lacunar strokes account for about 25 per cent of ischaemic strokes, which means that they account for roughly 20 per cent of all strokes. They may even occur 'silently' in that a person may not be aware of having had a stroke. In that sense they are more benign, in that the chances of surviving a lacunar stroke for at least a month is 95 per cent, as opposed to 85 per cent with other strokes. Also, 70 to 80 per cent of lacunar stroke survivors are functionally independent at one year.

A lacunar stroke is quite different from other strokes because the lacuna that is formed is deep inside the brain, inside the white matter. This will affect the wiring of the body but not mental or cognitive functioning.

Intra-cerebral-haemorrhagic stroke

These account for about 15 per cent of strokes. They occur when a blood vessel in the brain bursts and blood seeps into the brain tissue, causing damage. If the blood flow does not stop, this can be rapidly fatal.

A bleed into the brain can be utterly catastrophic, since there is not room for blood to collect and it forces its way into the tissue. How much it will bleed is not predictable and these strokes have a less good prognosis.

Subarachnoid haemorrhage

This accounts for up to 5 per cent of strokes, but tends to have a totally different presentation than other types of stroke.

It is the result of a bleed from an aneurysm, a sort of little balloon that forms on some brain vessels. The bleed in this case is between the arachnoid membrane and the pia membrane. These are two of the meninges (membranes) which cover the brain. (These membranes can become inflamed in meningitis, whether of viral or bacterial origin.)

Unlike most other strokes, which are relatively painless (see next chapter), a subarachnoid haemorrhage is usually associated with a sudden severe headache, as if something has exploded inside the head. Indeed, that is essentially what happens; an aneurysm bursts and blood oozes between the membranes.

The patient may retain consciousness or may slip into a coma. This sort of haemorrhage tends to occur in the young and the middle aged, so it is a different age group from most strokes. These aneurysms are often more common in some families and they may be congenital or present from birth.

A CT scan needs to be done urgently, and sometimes a lumbar puncture at the base of the spine will show blood in the cerebrospinal fluid. This is the fluid that bathes the brain and spinal cord.

Emergency treatment is vital, since there is a significant mortality rate of almost up to 50 per cent. Ten to fifteen per cent of patients die before reaching hospital and the mortality rate reaches as high as 40 per cent within the first week. Neurosurgery is occasionally necessary, although with modern advances in medicine it is possible sometimes to introduce coils into blood vessels, under radiological observation, to plug the bleeding vessel.

KEY POINTS

- If a cerebral aneurysm is present, the larger it is, the greater the chance of it bleeding.
- Many people have small berry aneurysms, which are less than 7 mm in diameter.
- The majority of aneurysms that burst are less than 1 cm in size.

Acute venous stroke

Up until now we have been looking at strokes that are the result of disruption of the arterial circulation to the brain – that is, of the vessels which carry blood from the heart to the brain. A much rarer type of stroke is one that affects the venous system, or the vessels that carry blood back from the brain to the heart.

This type of stroke is called a central venous sinus thrombosis and is the result of a clot blocking one of the dural venous sinuses which drain blood from the brain. The symptoms are often quite vague, but include headaches. Convulsions can occur, as can any of the general symptoms of stroke.

Diagnosis is by brain scan and the treatment is by the use of anticoagulants.

Other haemorrhages

These are not strokes as we know them, but they are conditions that can produce major problems and they always need to be considered in the diagnosis of stroke.

Extradural haemorrhage

This is a bleed following a head injury. It is usually from a fracture of the temporal bone at the temple of the skull and causes rupture of the middle meningeal artery.

This is the sort of injury that can occur in sport, when someone sustains a blow to the side of the head. There may be a lucid period when the individual just feels dazed, but some hours later there may be rapidly deepening wooziness followed by unconsciousness as the pressure inside the skull rises.

This is a neurosurgical emergency.

Subdural haemorrhage

This is a less dramatic picture. A subdural haemorrhage may also occur after a head injury; it is not a torrential bleed, however, but a slow ooze from smaller blood vessels in the subdural space, under the dura membrane, another of the meninges or membranes that covers the brain. The time lag between the injury and the onset of increasing drowsiness and headache can be as long as a week or even several weeks.

Urgent investigation and neurosurgery to evacuate the blood clot, which is called a haematoma, is needed.

Haemangioma rupture

This is similar to the spontaneous rupture of an aneurysm that occurs in subarachnoid haemorrhage, but it can be anywhere in the brain.

A haemangioma – or an arteriovenous malformation, as it is otherwise known – is a knot or collection of blood vessels. These can occur anywhere in the body and are potential sites that can rupture. If one occurs in the brain it can produce all of the symptoms and signs of a stroke.

Brain tumour

There are various types of tumour that can affect the brain. A primary brain tumour, or primary cerebral tumour, is one that arises inside the brain and is formed from some of the brain's own cells. It usually presents as a space-occupying lesion. This means that, as it grows, it gradually compresses part of the normal brain and may cause headaches or pressure effects on one or other of the cranial nerves. It is usually a much more gradual presentation than the dramatic onset of stroke.

Secondary cerebral tumours are tumours that have spread from a tumour somewhere else in the body, such as in cancer of the lung. The original tumour may be known about and may even have been treated. The secondary tumour may cause problems if it enlarges to encroach on structures within the brain, or it may mimic a stroke if there is a haemorrhage into the tumour.

In addition, a haemorrhage can occur into a cerebral tumour, to produce all of the symptoms of a stroke.

Cerebral infarction

The disruption to the supply of blood to part of the brain is only the start of the process. Within moments of oxygen deprivation a process called the ischaemic cascade begins. Effectively, because brain cells cannot store glucose the cells are unable to generate energy-carrying molecules and the vital functions of the cells stop. Sodium and calcium ions accumulate and cause the organelles, the components within the cells, to swell. At about six minutes the cells start to die and undergo a process called necrosis, which ultimately leads to scar formation called infarction.

If the blood supply is restored promptly, either naturally or as a result of clot-busting drugs, and recovery takes place within the first 24 hours, there will be no permanent damage.

If the ischaemia remains then the affected area will experience swelling and inflammation. This goes on for about a week.

Between one and four weeks the affected dead tissue, the infarcted area of tissue, will begin to change. It becomes soft and friable and may develop cysts to produce a functionally dead area of brain that is sponge-like. This sponge-like tissue is vulnerable to further damage from haemorrhage.

This really explains why the first month is a very important phase. Changes are still taking place in the brain which can impact on the recovery process. It is still a time to be cautious, since it is not certain at what stage of actual recovery the individual is at. A worsening of the swelling and local inflammation can produce a sudden worsening of the clinical condition.

One end point of an infarction is a lacuna, as described in the section on lacunar strokes earlier.

The outcome of a stroke

A stroke is a life-changing event, whether it is one from which the individual makes a total recovery or one from which one is left with a varying degree of disability.

The result after a stroke is dependent on the following factors:

- The cause of the stroke – whether it is ischaemic or haemorrhagic
- The type of stroke – which we shall cover in the next chapter
- How extensive the damage to the brain has been
- Which body functions have been affected by the stroke
- The speed and efficacy of the treatment.

There is a stark rule of thumb:

- One third of people who have a stroke make a full recovery
- One third recover with some permanent degree of disability
- One third die.

Regarding deaths from stroke:

- Ten per cent of all people who have a stroke die in the first week.

- Another 10 per cent of all people who have a stroke die in the first month.

- A further 10 per cent of all people who have a stroke die in the first year.

- People who have an ischaemic stroke have a better survival rate than those who have haemorrhagic strokes.

- Ischaemic strokes have a 15–45 per cent mortality at one month after the stroke.

- Haemorrhagic strokes have an 80 per cent mortality at one month after the stroke.

- Subarachnoid haemorrhages have up to 50 per cent mortality at one month after the event.

These figures may seem gloomy, but it is important to appreciate that stroke is a serious condition. The encouraging thing is that over 50 per cent of people who survive a stroke will be able to live at home and be able to function reasonably well, albeit perhaps with some disability. Others may need more extensive care; they will not be able to live independently, and will need help from one or more carers.

Complications of a stroke

By this we mean the sort of problems that can occur in the immediate aftermath of a stroke or which can develop over time.

- Aspiration of food or drink into the airway can occur if the swallowing mechanism has been disrupted. This is something that is checked on as a matter of urgency, since inhaled food can lead to choking and even asphyxiation. If it is actually aspirated into the lungs it can block off parts of the lung and lead to a dangerous condition called aspiration pneumonia.

- Loss of mobility can occur if the lower limbs are affected.

- Paralysis of any of the limbs can be permanent.

- Balance problems are common and can lead to increased falls and the dangers associated with them.

- Muscle spasticity is a huge potential problem and a large part of rehabilitation is aimed at getting muscles moving as much as possible.

- Difficulties with bladder and bowel control, which can be a major problem and can lead to other problems, such as increased frequency of urinary tract infections.

- Pressure sores in those stroke sufferers who are immobile.

- Difficulties with the various senses, especially vision.

- Nutritional problems if people have difficulty eating, perhaps necessitating parenteral nutrition (this means intravenous feeding).

- Difficulties with thinking, concentrating and remembering.

- Emotional disturbances are not uncommon. Anxiety, depression and mood swings can occur. This is most likely with strokes affecting the limbic system, which is in the midbrain.

- Personality changes and behavioural changes if the frontal lobe is affected.

- Difficulty with speech and communication. This can occur in different types of stroke.

- The risk of dementia may be increased.

It is also important to appreciate that there is an increased risk of having a second stroke in the first three months after a stroke, but after that the risk diminishes. It is important, of course, to adopt a lifestyle that reduces that risk; that means avoiding those habits that are injurious to one's health and those factors that make stroke more likely. We shall look at these in **Chapter 4, Risk factors for having a stroke and how to reduce your risk.**

The aim of stroke care is to act quickly with the appropriate investigation and treatment to reduce the death rate and reduce permanent disability.

KEY POINTS

Ischaemic strokes are more likely to occur in the areas supplied by the internal carotid arteries and the anterior and middle cerebral arteries. This is because they are quite convoluted in their pathways, which makes them more likely to 'silt up' with cholesterol.

A Transient Ischaemic Attack, sometimes called a mini-stroke, is caused by an obstruction rather than by haemorrhage.

Haemorrhagic strokes are more likely in the areas supplied by the vertebo-basilar system, since the vertebral arteries and the basilar artery are relatively straight, so they tend not to silt up.

Ischaemic strokes are almost always contralateral, meaning that they affect the opposite side of the body.

Haemorrhagic strokes may affect both sides of the body, since the bleed might damage both hemispheres of the brain.

Chapter 3

The different types of strokes

The functioning of the brain allows us to make sense of our world; we are able to move about and explore our environment, solve problems, communicate with others, appreciate beauty, read, write, enjoy music and have our various emotions stimulated. When we are well, we tend to take all of these things for granted. When someone experiences a stroke, some or all of these experiences may be taken away, creating a much more difficult and more hazardous world. Indeed, the individual may well become dependent on others for some or many aspects of life. It is important to appreciate this in the first instance, and to realise that brain attacks change lives.

In the last chapter we considered the mechanisms of strokes. Now we look at the different types of stroke. Essentially, these relate to which part of the brain has been affected by the blockage or the haemorrhage.

To recap, there are four parts of the brain, any of which can suffer damage from a stroke:

- Right hemisphere

- Left hemisphere

- Cerebellum

- Brain stem.

We shall look at the features one by one.

Which side – a source of confusion

People are often confused by the side that is affected. When one refers to either a right- or left-sided stroke, it refers to the side of the brain affected. On the other hand, when referring to the side of the body affected, the reference is to either a right- or a left-sided hemiplegia or hemiparesis.

Thus, a right-sided stroke refers to a blockage or bleed affecting the right side of the brain. It produces left-sided body symptoms, such as paralysis or partial paralysis.

It is for this reason that the old term 'cerebrovascular accident' (or CVA) is best avoided. People would refer to a right-sided CVA and sometimes be unsure whether it referred to the side of the bleed or the side of the body affected. Nowadays, we tend to describe the part of the brain affected.

Dominance

Most people have one hemisphere of the brain that is dominant. In the majority of right-handed people the left hemisphere is dominant. This tends to be the hemisphere which contains the speech centres, so if a right-handed person has a left hemisphere stroke they will experience speech problems and will have right side of body paralysis and sensory loss.

You would imagine that, similarly, the majority of naturally left-handed people would have a dominant right hemisphere. This is not always the case. About 50 per cent have dominance of the right and 50 per cent have dominance of the left hemisphere.

Right-hemisphere stroke

The right hemisphere controls and is responsible for:

- The movements of the left side of the body

- Analytical, judgement and perceptual tasks – e.g. assessing distance, speed, size and position.

A stroke affecting the right hemisphere may cause paralysis of the left side of the body. This is called a left-sided hemiplegia, when the whole of the left side is paralysed. It may also be called a left-sided hemiparesis. If only the left leg or arm is affected, it is called a partial hemiparesis.

Because of the right hemisphere's function in a person's sense of position, a right-hemisphere stroke survivor may have difficulty in judging distances or in assessing where their body or body parts are. Thus, they can have difficulty in reaching for objects, picking things up or doing fine movements such as buttoning clothes. They may also be more likely to fall or stumble.

Their perception of how things are arranged can also be distorted, so that they are unsure which is up and which is down. This can extend to reading and writing, so these abilities may become impaired.

This difficulty with judgement can spill over into the behavioural realm. Right-hemisphere survivors may develop a denial syndrome. They may not realise or forget that they have had a stroke or that they have any disability. As a result, they may become impulsive and lose awareness of their limitations. This seems to be because they forget that they have a problem. They may think that they can walk unaided, attempt fine movements that they do not have or become unaware of dangers of hot water, boiling liquids and hot objects.

They may also forget how to use their left side. In part, this can be the result of disturbance of the visual field. This is called left-sided neglect, and it results in the individual tending to neglect anything on the left side of the body. It is for this reason that a right-hemisphere stroke affecting the left side of the body can seem to cause a great deal of disability for the individual.

Memory problems are quite likely with right-hemisphere strokes. This is mainly the short-term memory that is affected.

Visual problems are more common in right-hemisphere strokes. We shall consider this further in **Chapter 8, Complications after a stroke.**

KEY POINTS

Right-hemisphere syndrome is a term used to describe the collection of symptoms and difficulties that arise from damage to the right hemisphere of the brain. Damage could be from various causes including a right-hemisphere stroke.

In general, it seems that a stroke in the right hemisphere can be more disabling, because the right hemisphere organises how things are judged and assessed. It seems to be more dominant in many cognitive functions. To put it simply, the brain of a right-hemisphere stroke survivor seems to forget how to put things together, so that the person seems to fail to understand what they are experiencing.

Communication is often impaired, but not in the same way as with left-hemisphere stroke. It is more to do with failure to understand and process speech.

The following areas of difficulty can arise:

- Attention and inability to concentrate
- Left-sided neglect
- Denial of problem
- Behavioural change and emotional ability
- Memory problems
- Disorientation about dates and time
- Problem-solving difficulty
- Reasoning difficulty
- Communication problems – e.g. loss of humour, failure to appreciate nuances, inappropriate speech.

Left-hemisphere stroke

The left hemisphere controls and is responsible for:

- The movement of the right side of the body

- Speech, language understanding and writing ability.

A stroke affecting the left hemisphere may cause paralysis of the right side of the body. When the whole of the right side is paralysed, this is called a right-sided hemiplegia. It may also be called a right-sided hemi-paresis or, if only the leg or the arm is affected, a partial hemi-paresis.

Speech difficulties are common in left-hemisphere stroke survivors. This is mainly because the left hemisphere contains the speech centres, Broca's area and Wernicke's area, so disturbance in their function can affect the individual's ability to both interpret and understand language and to produce speech.

Dysphasia or aphasia are the names given to speech disorders. Aphasia means 'no speech' and dysphasia means 'difficulty with speech'. The two words are often used interchangeably. They can occur in other conditions, such as with brain tumours, brain infections and in dementia conditions such as Alzheimer's disease. About a third of all stroke survivors will experience some difficulty with speech.

Dysarthria is another problem that can occur when the muscles used to produce speech have been affected.

Left-hemisphere stroke survivors tend to become more cautious than right-hemisphere stroke survivors, who become impulsive.

They may seem to take longer to process information and may need repetition of information.

Memory problems may become apparent, as with right-hemisphere stroke survivors.

Cerebellar stroke

The cerebellum is the control box for information that is transmitted from all over the body about where our body parts are at any time. It controls reflexes and balance and helps you to maintain coordination. A stroke in this area can be very disabling.

Brain-stem stroke

Theses strokes can have a catastrophic effect. The brain stem is where all of the body's automatic mechanisms are operated, which includes the ability to breathe, pump the heart and maintain the internal environment of the body, such as blood pressure and digestive function.

Locked-in syndrome

This is the name given to a severe brain-stem stroke. It occurs in about 1 per cent of all strokes and is a state of complete paralysis such that the patient is unable to move or communicate verbally. All of the voluntary muscles are paralysed, except for the eyes. There is complete awareness, however. It is as if the individual is locked in their own head and unable to communicate with others.

A more severe variant is 'totally locked-in syndrome' in which even the eye muscles are paralysed. The condition is also known as cerebro-medullo-spinal disconnection, pseudocoma or ventral pontine syndrome.

The cause may be a stroke affecting the basilar artery, the main artery that supplies the back part of the Circle of Willis.

There have been some high-profile cases in the UK in which locked-in stroke survivors have campaigned for the right to have assisted dying. At the time of writing the legal situation remains unchanged, and euthanasia is not legal in the UK.

Living will

It would seem appropriate to mention this here. Many people want to make their wishes known about treatment that they would like to refuse should they be unable to communicate in the future. This is commonly called a Living Will, but it is in fact a bit misleading, since it has nothing to do with money or property, as with a will. More correctly it is called an 'Advance Decision'.

Under ordinary circumstances, if you fall ill there will be an opportunity to discuss treatment with your doctor. If, however, you are suddenly taken ill and admitted to hospital when unconscious and unable to communicate your wishes, then the medical team will try to use all means to save your life. If this is not what you would wish, for example if you had a stroke and were unable to communicate, then you might consider making an Advance Decision.

This is a notification on paper that in certain circumstances you would wish to refuse certain types of treatment. This could include resuscitation, or it may be a desire not to be given intravenous drugs, a blood transfusion or parenteral feeding.

An Advance Decision is legally binding in England and Wales. Medical and nursing professionals must accept your decision, regardless of their own opinions. It cannot be revoked by the family. The situation is different in Scotland and Northern Ireland.

Sometimes the term 'Advance Statement' is used, but this is not quite the same thing. Whereas the Advance Decision is a refusal of treatment, an Advance Statement is an expression of the individual's desires. It may relate to food preferences and religious or philosophical beliefs. It is not legally binding.

KEY POINTS

- An Advance Decision is notification of a refusal to have treatment, should the individual be unable to communicate to medical professionals.

- An Advance Decision can be made by anyone over the age of 18, who is of sound mind.

- It is a legal document that cannot be overruled by the family or medical or nursing staff.

- The individual who made it can revoke it at any time.

- Doctors and family should be aware that an Advance Decision has been made.

- Age UK have helpful factsheets that can be downloaded here: www.ageuk.org.uk/health-wellbeing/

  Age UK, Tavis House, 1–6 Tavistock Square, London WC1H 9NA. Telephone for advice: 0800 169 6565

Mini-strokes

A mini-stroke or, more correctly, a Transient Ischaemic Attack, is a brain attack, the symptoms of which quickly resolve within 24 hours. The name 'ischaemic' indicates that this is the result of a blockage, rather than a bleed.

It is, however, important not to think that the term 'mini-stroke' is a reason to be complacent. A mini-stroke is a serious matter and it must always be acted upon in the same way as a stroke. That means dealing with it as a medical emergency and not waiting to see what happens. The fact is that 20–30 per cent of people who have a TIA will go on to have a full stroke at some stage, and 5 per cent of people who have a TIA will have a stroke within two days.

We shall return to the important business of assessment and investigation of TIA in **Chapter 5, When a stroke strikes.**

Chapter 4

Risk factors for having a stroke and how to reduce your risk

The important thing to appreciate is that a stroke is essentially both a preventable and a treatable condition. As we have seen so far, it can have a devastating effect on the stroke survivor, but it can also have a far-reaching effect upon a family.

If a stroke has occurred in your family then you should consider taking steps to reduce your risk of having a stroke. It is of course sensible for everyone to try to reduce their risk.

Some of the following risk factors cannot be altered, yet many others can. First of all, let us look at those factors that you cannot control.

Risks you cannot control

Your genetic make-up

Some families seem to have more strokes than others. There may be something in their genes that predisposes certain people.

Having said that, there are no readily available tests that can predict whether one will have a stroke; indeed, it may be that the families with a higher incidence of strokes have other factors that something could be done about. For example, they may have a diet that puts them at risk or they may smoke or drink excessively.

The simple fact is that if you do have a family that has a higher incidence of stroke, you should see your doctor to have your overall risk rated, and then you should try to reduce your risk from the factors that you can do something about.

There is a rare inherited genetic disorder called 'Cerebral autosomal dominant arteriopathy with subcortical infarcts and leukoencephalopathy', usually referred to as CADASIL. It is a condition associated with frequent migraines and repeated strokes. It starts at a young age, around 30.

It can be diagnosed by blood and tissue sampling. There is no specific treatment, but antiplatelet drugs like aspirin, clopidogrel and dipyridamole may be used to reduce the risk of having a stroke.

Age

Strokes can occur at any age, even – rarely – in babies. Strokes do seem to be more common as one ages, with most strokes occurring after the age of 55 years. Thereafter, the risk increases gradually. The reason seems to be the increasing likelihood of atherosclerosis as one ages.

A study in 2012 from the University of Cincinnati College of Medicine in Ohio looked at stroke rates in people aged between 20 and 54 years of age in greater Cincinnati and northern Kentucky. Looking at data collected about first strokes from the early 1900s until 2005 showed that the proportion of first strokes under the age of 55 years increased in that time from 13 per cent to 19 per cent. Over the same period, the average age of having a first stroke fell from 71 years to 60 years of age.

Those are worrying statistics, because one possible reason is that people's lifestyles are changing, as the incidence of obesity and diabetes are increasing.

Gender

Males generally have a higher risk than females, although in middle age there is a slight increased risk for women over men. It seems that this relates to hormonal change around the menopause, and possibly to the fact that women may be taking hormone replacement therapy (HRT) during the menopause.

Ethnic background

Strokes occur in all ethnic backgrounds, but people of African, African-Caribbean or South Asian origin are at increased risk.

ETHRISK

The ETHRISK (Ethnic group CHD Risk Calculator) is the name for a test tool that can be used to calculate the risk of heart disease and stroke risk in British black and minority ethnic groups. It is used for people aged 35–74 years, without diabetes or a past history of cerebro-vascular disease. It is based on sex, age, systolic blood pressure, cholesterol levels and smoking status.

Your general practitioner will be able to discuss this, if requested.

Risks you can control

The following are factors that are important and for which there is usually something that can be done.

Hypertension

Uncontrolled high blood pressure or hypertension is the biggest risk factor for stroke. It is sensible for all adults to have their blood pressure recorded at least once every year, since it is an insidious condition that can creep up on an individual without them having any symptoms whatsoever. People often assume that headaches will be the first symptom but, more often than not, it is symptomless.

Blood pressure is the force of blood against the walls of arteries and is recorded as two numbers: firstly, the systolic pressure, which represents the pressure attained as the heart beats; secondly, the diastolic pressure, which represents the pressure in the circulation as the heart relaxes between beats. The measurement is written with the systolic figure on top and the diastolic number on the bottom. These numbers each represent the recorded pressure in mmHg (mm of mercury, which is the standard means of measuring pressure).

Hypertension, or high blood pressure, affects about a billion people worldwide. In the UK, the prevalence of hypertension has been estimated to be 42 per cent in people aged 35–64. Preventing high blood pressure is well worthwhile in order to reduce one's future risk of heart attack, stroke or kidney disease.

It is currently recommended that a level of 135/85 or less is the level that should be aimed at.

To put the risk into figures, each rise of 2 mmHg of systolic pressure increases the risk of increased mortality from heart disease by 7 per cent, and of increased mortality from stroke by 10 per cent. Keeping the blood pressure controlled, therefore, is the single most important thing to do to reduce the risk of stroke.

Salt intake

I mention this here, since one's salt intake may have a direct bearing on blood pressure.

The fact is that salt helps to push blood pressure up by somehow affecting internal regulatory mechanisms that push the pressure higher. It is important to appreciate that blood pressure is very important. It is a real risk factor for strokes, heart failure and heart attacks. Sodium seems to be the culprit, and since salt is the main source of sodium in the diet it is the obvious thing to reduce to minimise the risk.

Adults are advised to consume no more than 6 g of salt a day – that is, about a teaspoon. The average intake in the UK is about 9 g, or about 50 per cent more than is recommended. And for a large number of people who already have raised blood pressure that is very significant.

When you look at labels, don't be fooled if they only give the sodium content. To get the actual salt level, multiply it by 2.5.

Smoking

The smoking habit has no health benefits whatsoever, but greatly increases the risk of developing many potentially lethal conditions, including stroke.

Basically, someone who smokes at all is twice as likely as a non-smoker to sustain a stroke. This is an increase in both ischaemic strokes and haemorrhagic strokes.

A study from South Korea, published in the *Journal of Neurology, Neurosurgery and Psychiatry* in 2012, compared 426 people who had a haemorrhagic stroke with 426 people who had not had a stroke. They found that 38 per cent of people who had a brain bleed were current smokers, compared with 24 per cent of the non-bleed controls. They also found that smokers who had a brain haemorrhage could reduce their risk of having a further stroke by 60 per cent over five years by stopping smoking.

Passive smoking also increases the risk of stroke. It has been shown that living with a smoker and inhaling their used smoke regularly can increase the risk of a stroke in a non-smoking, 'passive smoker' by up to 80 per cent. This is part of the reason for the ban on smoking in public spaces that is gradually coming into effect in more countries around the world.

Obesity

It is known that increasing levels of obesity are associated with increased incidence of stroke. It seems likely that being obese increases the individual's risk, yet it is not known for sure whether it is the obesity itself or other secondary factors that increase the risk. Secondary risk factors include diabetes, raised cholesterol and possibly, hypertension. Nonetheless, as a marker of good health, it is advisable to keep one's weight to a recommended level.

The early death rate of people who are 30–40 lb overweight is 30 per cent greater than one would expect in a general population of people of normal weight. More alarmingly, there is a 50 per cent increase in early death for men who weigh more than 40 per cent above ideal body weight.

Ideally you should aim for a Body Mass Index of 25. Body Mass Index is an accepted means of relating weight to height. It is easily worked out by dividing the weight in kilograms by the square of the height in metres. It is essentially giving an estimation of the human body fat, although it does not actually measure fat.

Alcohol

Drinking alcohol is not in itself a risk. Indeed, moderate alcohol intake may have a beneficial effect on one's health. Excessive intake, however, is a definite risk for having a stroke.

The Royal College of Physicians recommends that men should not drink more than 21 units of alcohol a week, and women 14 units a week. It is suggested that, for sensible drinking, the daily alcohol intake should not exceed 3–4 units for men or 2–3 units for women. Continued drinking at the upper limit is not advised, and at least two alcohol-free days a week should be taken, particularly after heavy drinking. As a rule of thumb, heavy drinking is defined as 6 units in six hours.

A unit is either a small measure of spirits, a small glass of wine or a half pint of beer or lager.

Binge drinking is a real risk because it can push the blood pressure up quite quickly. It also has secondary effects from the breakdown products of alcohol, which include the toxic effects of aldehydes, which can have a deleterious effect upon the liver. In addition, binge drinking often makes individuals lose their inhibitions and their control, so that they may eat more, do foolhardy things or even end up vomiting and causing a rise in pressure that can be transmitted up to a blood vessel in the brain, exceeding its ability to sustain the pressure. Stroke could be the consequence.

A study from France in 2012 published in the journal *Neurology* looked at the drinking habits of 540 patients who had experienced an intracerebral haemorrhage. They found that one quarter were heavy drinkers, consuming at least four drinks a day. Their haemorrhages occurred earlier than non-drinkers in the group, with an average age of 60 years when they had their stroke, as opposed to 74 years for the non-drinkers.

Inactivity

This is really quite a commonsense thing. The less active a person is, the less fit they are likely to be. They are then more likely to put on weight and to lose the tone in their muscles. It becomes a vicious circle.

The benefits of regular exercise are well known in terms of helping to reduce the risk of various ailments, including stroke. For one thing, it helps to control weight, it helps to reduce cholesterol and it reduces the risk of developing diabetes.

In terms of losing weight, people often think that its value is simply a matter of burning calories. It is not as simple as that. Exercise has quite a profound effect on the body by virtue of what it does to the metabolism. Exercise seems to stimulate a hormone called 'irisin'. It is named after Iris, the Greek messenger goddess, because it seems to deliver a message from the muscles that stimulates these amazing changes in the body.

Scientists found this hormone in the membranes of muscle cells when they were investigating a particular gene. They were aware that exercise somehow switched this gene on. Having found the hormone, they used lab cultures and mice to show that irisin has a powerful effect on white adipose tissue. This is the type of fat that accumulates under the skin and contributes to obesity. The irisin causes the body to convert white fat to brown fat. Brown fat is regarded as 'good' fat, because it actually burns off more calories than exercise alone. Brown fat produces heat by burning calories. Indeed, it produces 300 times more heat than any organ in the body.

In the mice studies the researchers found that not only was white fat converted into brown fat, but it had a positive effect on glucose tolerance. This could be of vital importance as a treatment in the future, since the link between obesity and diabetes is well known.

In practical terms, it is worth incorporating exercise into your day. This does not have to mean going to a gym; you can do it simply by walking more. A study from Missouri looked at the effect of short bursts of exercise on a group of men and women who did not regularly exercise. Over the trial period, on three occasions they were given a high-fat meal, consisting of a milkshake with heavy whipping cream. Before one of the meals they exercised vigorously for 30 minutes. Another time they exercised for three 10-minute sessions. On the last occasion they did not exercise. Interestingly, the short bursts of activity, equivalent to three brisk 10-minute walks, had the best effect in lowering the blood fat levels.

Cholesterol

Most people know that a high cholesterol level in the blood is not good for you. It can increase the risk of heart disease or of having a stroke. It is not just the level of cholesterol that matters, however, but the relative balance between good cholesterol and bad cholesterol. Essentially, the lower the level of bad cholesterol the lower is your risk.

Cholesterol is a type of waxy, fat substance that is found in all of the cells of the body. It is in fact an important substance for the body, but you just don't want too much of it. Cholesterol is carried around the bloodstream in packets called lipoproteins. The lipo is the inside part of the package and consists of fat; the protein is the outer part. There are two types of lipoprotein which carry your cholesterol: low density lipoprotein or LDL, commonly known as the bad cholesterol, and high density lipoprotein or HDL, commonly thought of as good cholesterol.

The problem with too much LDL cholesterol is that it tends to cause a build-up of cholesterol in your artery walls. Imagine that the lining of an artery is like a sponge with lots of small holes in it. Think of the LDL cholesterol as being like a small ball, about the size of the holes in the sponge. By contrast, HDL cholesterol is like a much bigger ball, much larger than the holes. So, if you have blood carrying a mixture of both types of ball a large proportion of the small balls will lodge in the holes. The larger ones will just bounce off and carry on their way. That is how bad cholesterol affects your blood vessels.

Recent research from the USA has shown that when people eat cholesterol-lowering foods in addition to going on a low-fat diet they can reduce the bad cholesterol by 13 per cent, as opposed to a mere 3 per cent when they only reduce the fat content. The beneficial foods are those containing plant sterols, such as nuts and foods with viscous fibre, such as barley, oats and soy protein as in soya milk, tofu and soy meat substitutes.

If the cholesterol level is found to be high then one should do all that one can to reduce it. There are various dietary things which may help, as can exercise, but many people will require one of the statin group of drugs. We shall consider this in **Chapter 7, Medication**.

Other medical conditions

There are several conditions which predispose people to having strokes, so their management becomes all the more important. We have already considered hypertension. This is the most important medical condition that increases the risk of having a stroke.

Atrial fibrillation

Atrial fibrillation is the name given to a condition characterised by an irregular heartbeat. Because of this irregularity, clots can form within the heart that may be pumped around the body to lodge in a brain artery.

The heart has four chambers. In atrial fibrillation the two upper chambers, called atria (from the Latin *atrium*, meaning entrance hall) do not beat in harmony with the rest of the heart, but quiver. As a result, the overall function of the heart becomes less efficient and the heart may start to fail, the result being that the individual gets short of breath.

Because the atria do not effectively pump the blood out, the blood inside them becomes sluggish – this makes clot formation more likely. This happens more often in the left atrium, so a clot can easily be flicked out into the blood supply to the brain.

Atrial fibrillation is most common after the age of 65 years and is usually a result of some degree of atherosclerosis causing coronary artery disease.

It can also occur at younger ages in people with advanced uncontrolled hypertension, in hyperthyroidism (overactive thyroid), after a heart attack, in people with problems associated with the mitral valve of the heart and in a variety of lung disorders, including emphysema. Some heart conditions can be congenital, meaning that they are present from birth. If a medical examination reveals the presence of a murmur then it should be precisely diagnosed, possibly involving a referral to a specialist.

KEY POINTS

- Between 2 and 4 per cent of people with atrial fibrillation without a history of TIA or of stroke will have a major stroke within a year.

- If they go on to have a TIA, then their risk increases to 20–30 per cent.

- There are 50,000 new cases of atrial fibrillation each year in the UK

- 1 in 200 people aged 50–60 years have atrial fibrillation.

- 1 in 10 people over 80 years have atrial fibrillation.

Atrial fibrillation should be treated, either to try to revert the heart into a normal rhythm, or by the use of medication to reduce the chance of the blood clotting.

Past medical history

If someone has a previous history of TIA or of stroke then they are at increased risk of having a stroke at some stage. Of those people who have had a TIA, 20–30 per cent will go on to have a stroke.

Diabetes mellitus

Diabetes is a disorder of metabolism in which a person has high blood sugar. This can be either because insulin production by the pancreas is inadequate or because the body cells no longer respond to it. The main symptoms of diabetes are increased thirst and frequent desire to pass urine.

The condition was known to the ancient Egyptians and the ancient Greeks. Indeed, the second-century physician Arateus introduced the name diabetes, meaning 'siphon', because of the fact that people drank lots of water and seemed to siphon it through their system.

Dr Thomas Willis – the physician to King Charles II who discovered the Circle of Willis discussed in Chapter 2 which is so important in our understanding about strokes – discovered that the urine of diabetic people tasted sweet. It was he who added the second name, 'mellitus', from the Latin for honey.

There are three types of diabetes:

Type 1 diabetes – which used to be called 'juvenile diabetes' because it tended to occur acutely in childhood or adolescence. This is an auto-immune condition in which the immune system attacks the insulin-producing cells in the pancreas. There is therefore a deficiency of insulin and the individual will have to take insulin injections for the rest of their life. It accounts for 10 per cent of the cases of diabetes.

Type 2 diabetes – where the body does not produce enough insulin or the cells of the body fail to recognise and react to it. This used to be called maturity-onset diabetes and accounts for about 90 per cent of cases of diabetes.

It is more common the older one becomes and, the more overweight a person is, the more it is likely to develop. It necessitates control either through diet, or through diet and oral medication with various hypoglycaemic or blood-sugar-lowering drugs.

Gestational diabetes – is diabetes that starts during pregnancy. It has to be controlled since the unborn child will be put at risk.

Diabetes is an independent risk factor for stroke and heart disease. This means that even when one allows for the fact that obesity, raised cholesterol and hypertension are more common in diabetes, when they are all controlled the risk is still double that of a non-diabetic person. This makes it all the more important for diabetics to do all that they can to keep their sugar levels under control.

KEY POINTS

- Diabetes at least doubles the risk of having a stroke.
- Diabetes accounts for 10–20 per cent of strokes.

Blood disorders

There are various blood problems that make a stroke more likely. Generally, these are conditions in which the viscosity (thickness) of the blood is increased; this makes clot formation likely.

Sickle cell disease

This is an inherited blood disease characterised by sickle-shaped red blood cells. It is most common in people from the tropics or sub-tropics where malaria is prevalent. And since it is an inherited trait, it can occur in people whose ancestry stretches back to that part of the world.

Up to 25 per cent of people with this condition will have a stroke before the age of 45 years.

Factor V Leiden gene

This is not a disease, but the presence of a particular gene. Factor V is a clotting factor in the blood. People who have Factor V deficiency will bleed more easily. On the other hand, people with Factor V Leiden have an increased tendency to clot their blood. In the UK, 5 per cent of the population have one or more of the genes for Factor V Leiden.

Myeloproliferative disorders

These are a group of blood conditions in which the numbers of blood cells are increased, resulting in increased 'coagulability' of the blood. Examples are polycythemia vera and essential thrombocytosis.

Migraine

It used to be thought that migraine was merely a condition that caused painful headaches. It is caused by spasm and dilation of the blood vessels in the scalp and the brain. However, research published in the *American Journal of Medicine* in 2010 analysed the results of 21 previous studies on migraine and stroke. It concluded that people with migraine have twice the risk of having a stroke than those who do not suffer from migraine.

This really means that, if you are a migraine sufferer, then you should be extra determined to control your risk factors for stroke; you should not smoke or binge drink, and you should keep your weight under control.

Inflammatory conditions

There are various conditions which cause inflammation of blood vessels and, as a result, the build-up of blood clots becomes more likely. Temporal arteritis, a condition causing inflammation of the arteries in the scalp and skull, is known to be associated with stroke and treatment is needed urgently with steroids to reduce the inflammation and keep it under control.

The condition of systemic lupus erythematosus also increases the risk of stroke.

Rheumatoid arthritis and psoriasis

A Danish study[1] suggests that patients with rheumatoid arthritis (RA) have a 40 per cent increased risk of atrial fibrillation and a 30 per cent increased risk of stroke compared with those without RA.

The same research team also suggest that psoriasis sufferers may also have an increased risk. In both cases, it is a good reason to minimise other risk factors.

Drugs

Some drugs are associated with an increased risk of stroke; anticoagulants, for example, are associated with an increased risk of haemorrhagic stroke. The oral contraceptive pill is associated with an increased risk of blood clot formation, and therefore of ischaemic stroke. The risk seems to be greater the older the woman is and the higher the oestrogen content of the pill.

HRT or hormone replacement therapy may be associated with an increased risk of ischaemic stroke.

Some over-the-counter drugs, including cough and cold remedies containing drugs belonging to the group of drugs called sympathomimetics (e.g. pseudoephedrine and phenylephrine), may increase the risk slightly, if taken regularly and especially by people with other risk factors such as hypertension.

Recreational drugs like cocaine and amphetamines may be associated with haemorrhagic stroke. This can occur in younger patients with an aneurysm that was not previously known about.

Pregnancy

It is not usual for young women to have strokes, but pregnancy increases the risk about ten times compared with non-pregnant women because enormous physiological changes come about during pregnancy. For the vast majority of women the risk still remains small, and only about 1 in every 3,000 pregnancies will be complicated by a stroke. This is more likely if the woman develops a condition called pre-eclampsia, which is associated with a drastic rise in blood pressure.

Diet

Studies have shown that a Mediterranean diet reduces the risk of cardiovascular events such as heart attacks and strokes. This reduction in risk can be by as much as 50 per cent.[2] It seems to come about by reducing the lipid content in the blood and also by producing a beneficial effect on blood sugars. It seems to reduce insulin resistance, one of the problems that leads to diabetes.

Chapter 5

When a stroke strikes

It can be a terrifying event when you are with someone who has a stroke. Imagine how much more alarming it must be for them when they suddenly experience loss of functioning of parts of their body – or worse, if they suddenly lose consciousness and then regain it some time later only to find that they cannot move parts of their body or are unable to communicate.

There is no typical stroke. There are many variants, depending upon which part of the brain has been affected, as we saw in **Chapter 3, The different types of stroke**. The most important thing to appreciate is that a stroke is a medical emergency. It is vital to get help for yourself if you think you are having a stroke, or for someone you are with who seems to be having a stroke. Speed is essential.

You do not need to diagnose what sort of stroke someone is having; that is up to the medical staff who will see the patient. What you need to recognise is whether a stroke is occurring.

The FAST test

The Stroke Association is running a campaign which you may have seen on television or on posters or in magazines and newspapers. It is a simple mnemonic, which alerts you to the things to look for and the action you must take.

FAST stands for:

FACIAL weakness – ask the person to smile. Look to see if the mouth is drooping on one side.

ARM weakness – can the person raise both arms?

SPEECH problems – can the person speak clearly, without slurring? Do they understand what you are saying?

TIME to call – the emergency number for medical assistance.

Quite simply, if the person fails any of these tests there is enough evidence to suspect that they are having a stroke. The faster that you get help, the better the prospect of minimising damage to their brain. This will improve their chances of recovery. It may even save their life.

Why mini-strokes must be treated seriously

Mini-strokes, or Transient Ischaemic Attacks (TIAs), must not be regarded as insignificant. These are brain attacks, which are reversible and clear up within 24 hours, but are just as important to recognise, investigate and treat as are full-blown strokes.

They must never be ignored. People may be tempted to just wait and see if the symptoms disappear, but one can never be sure whether it is a TIA or a stroke that is developing and getting worse.

Precious time may be wasted by delaying. If the FAST test described above is positive, then it is time to call for urgent help.

Also, even if there has been a cluster of symptoms that have reversed themselves, they should still be chtute ecked out by a doctor. The thing is that, although a TIA has been reversed, it could be followed by a much more severe and even life-threatening stroke.

KEY POINTS

- 20–30 per cent of people who have a TIA will go on to have a full stroke at some stage.
- 5 per cent of people who have a TIA will have a stroke within 2 days.
- 10–15 per cent of people who have a TIA will have a stroke within 3 months.

Obviously, most people are immediately relieved when they find out that their symptoms have all reversed and they are told that they have had a mini-stroke. The name makes it sound a lot less significant than a stroke. Indeed, it minimises the impact of the event in the patient's mind. However, not all mini-strokes or TIAs have the same significance and it is an important function of the stoke unit to fully assess the TIA and work out the relative risk of having a further stroke.

The goal of TIA management is, of course, to prevent the occurrence of a further stroke.

Assessing the risk of having a major stroke

After a TIA has been confirmed, it is important to assess the risk of having a stroke. The $ABCD^2$ algorithm is one method that is commonly used as recommended by NICE (National Institute for Health and Clinical Excellence).

It stands for:

Age

Blood pressure

Clinical features of symptoms

Duration of TIA

Diabetes – whether present or not

On the basis of these five factors a score is obtained that allows the risk of a stroke within the following two days to be calculated.

Age – if 60 or above – 1 point

Blood pressure – systolic pressure 140 or above or diastolic pressure 90 or above – 1 point

Clinical features – one-sided weakness with or without speech impairment – 2 points OR speech impairment without one-sided weakness – 1 point

Duration of TIA – 60 minutes or more – 2 points

   or 10–59 minutes – 1 point

Diabetes – absent – 0 points

Diabetes – present – 1 point

Research has shown that the higher the ABCD^2 score, the greater the risk of stroke. The risk value seems to be constant to the figure at 2 days, 7 days, 30 days and 90 days, so it is a valuable test.[3]

ABCD^2 Score	2-day risk	Recommendation
0–3	1.0%	Hospital observation unnecessary in absence of other risks like atrial fibrillation
4–5	4.1%	Hospital observation justified
6–7	8.1%	Hospital observation worthwhile

NICE recommends that, after a TIA, a patient should be started on daily aspirin (300 mg) daily and secondary prevention begun for other risk factors such as blood pressure, cholesterol and diabetes, as well as advice given about lifestyle, such as weight control and stopping smoking.

With low ABCD^2 scores, specialist assessment and investigations including brain imaging should take place within a week. With high scores or with crescendo TIAs (meaning having two or more TIAs in a week), such investigation should take place within 24 hours.

Assess the carotid arteries

Part of the assessment of someone who has had a stroke or a non-disabling stroke is to determine the calibre and patency of the carotid arteries. These are found in the front of the neck and supply the front part of the Circle of Willis, the circulation to the brain; narrowing here may be the cause of a TIA or of a stroke.

The physical examination may reveal a 'bruit', the sound of turbulence in the flow of blood through the carotid artery on one or both sides of the neck. This is picked up by the doctor listening to the neck through a stethoscope.

A carotid Doppler, a duplex scan and an angiogram may be ordered. The angiogram is a special X-ray in which a radiopaque dye (meaning it shows up on X-ray as cloudiness) is injected into a blood vessel via a special catheter that is threaded all the way up to the carotid artery from the femoral artery in the groin.

The dye is followed under X-ray, and if there is narrowing of the neck vessels or the cerebral vessels it will show up on the angiogram.

If there is significant disease in the carotid arteries then surgery may be an option. It is a procedure that actually carries a real risk of producing a stroke, so it will be offered only to people with a very marked narrowing and therefore a high risk of having a stroke in the next few years. This operation is called a carotid endarterectomy. An alternative is to do an angioplasty, in which a tiny balloon is inserted by a catheter and inflated to attempt to open up the narrowed vessel. A stent is then inserted during the procedure to keep the vessel open.

Huge variation in the clinical picture

Although we can explain many of the symptoms that people experience when they have a stroke, no-one can predict exactly what is going to happen when someone starts to develop a symptom.

One stroke can cause fairly minimal symptoms from which a complete recovery is made within hours (as in TIAs); others can take a few days or weeks and yet others can be catastrophic and cause collapse and instant death. In general:

Ischaemic strokes can be fast or slow to develop. Symptoms may progress gradually as the ischaemic area undergoes swelling and inflammation, so that the extent of the stroke is not immediately apparent. This is often called a stroke in evolution, since the stroke is continuing to evolve.

Haemorrhagic strokes are sudden. They are more likely to be associated with a headache, as they are caused by a burst blood vessel. And they are more likely to be catastrophic than ischaemic strokes.

Subarachnoid haemorrhages are sudden, with severe headache as if something has exploded. They are also associated with meningism. This refers to signs associated with irritation of the meninges, the membranes that surround the brain. There will be intense tenderness and discomfort on moving the head off the pillow.

The symptoms of stroke

There are many possibilities, depending upon which parts of the brain have been affected. They can occur without the individual even having any awareness that they have had a stroke. Someone may notice that they just seem off balance, or that their mouth is drooping or an eyelid is drooping. Pain may or may not be a feature.

Headaches

A headache may, however, be associated and the pattern of the headache may be significant. Any sudden severe headache is suspicious if the individual has never previously had headaches. If it occurs when the person is lying down, possibly even being woken from sleep with a headache, then it is suspicious and should be acted upon, which means seeking immediate medical advice. Finally, if the headache is worse when the person turns the head, bends over or strains when coughing or when trying to open the bowel, then medical advice should be sought.

Weakness of any limb or of one side of the body

If a limb simply will not work then the possibility of a stroke needs to be considered urgently. Difficulty walking when there was no previous difficulty is highly significant, as is an inability to raise both arms, which is why it is a component of the FAST test.

There may be obvious weakness of one side of the body or of one side of the face. The lip may droop on one side.

Level of consciousness

It is an absolute medical emergency if a person suddenly collapses and goes into a coma. They should be put into the recovery position and medical help should be sought. If they seem drowsy or inexplicably intoxicated then that could also be an early symptom.

Slurring speech

If this occurs out of the blue it may be significant and the FAST test should be applied.

Sudden loss of balance

This can be slight and the person may just tend to veer in one direction when they are walking, or it can be so severe that they feel dizzy and fall over. It could be a sign of a cerebellar stroke.

Loss of coordination

This may present itself as sudden clumsiness, knocking into things or knocking things over. Or it could be a sudden inability to perform a normal task like picking up a book or a cup.

Inability to swallow

The inability to swallow or sudden unexplained choking is highly suggestive and medical help should be sought immediately. No further drink or food should be given or taken until it is demonstrated that you can swallow. This can be a danger symptom.

Sudden difficulty with vision

Any sudden loss of vision always has to be investigated urgently. There are many patterns of visual difficulty that can occur and we shall consider them in **Chapter 8, Complications after a stroke**.

A quite marked visual loss may not always be apparent to the individual, especially if there has been a right-hemisphere stroke.

Alteration in any sense

Suddenly experiencing a bizarre taste or smell, or being aware of a change in hearing may not have anything to do with a stroke but, if coupled with any other physical symptom, it is as well to be checked.

Altered sensation

Any sudden numbness or inability to feel when you touch something, or you are touched but fail to feel it, or failure to feel pain or altered temperature (for example, not being aware of a burn), should be investigated.

Loss of bladder or bowel control

This is a common feature of a stroke in someone who has always had control of their functions.

Sudden memory problems

This can be a feature of several neurological conditions, but a stroke has to be at the top of the list. It is usually a significant memory loss, even amounting to amnesia or loss of memory for where they are or even who they are. Minor degrees of memory loss may not be so apparent, yet can be significant.

Reading and writing

Sometimes a stroke can suddenly impair someone's ability to perform these tasks. They may not even be able to read or write their own name.

Sudden mood or personality change

If a person is subject to rapid changes of mood then it may not be significant, but if they exhibit a sudden uncharacteristic and inexplicable alteration in mood or behaviour, then this could indicate that something has happened in the brain. For example:

- Sudden violent outburst of temper in the normally placid

- Sudden foul language in the normally softly-spoken

- Extreme tearfulness in the usually cheerful.

Initial assessment

Nowadays, it may often be a paramedic who performs the initial professional assessment, if the FAST test has been applied and an ambulance has been called. On the other hand, if the person has attended at their GP's surgery then the doctor will perform a physical examination; if there is a suspicion of a stroke it is likely that an admission to hospital will be arranged straight away for further investigation.

Not everyone with a stroke will be admitted to hospital. For instance, some elderly people in a residential or nursing home, who are extremely frail or who are suffering already from a terminal condition, may choose to remain where they are.

No-one will be forced to undergo admission and treatment against their will, but if admission seems to be in the individual's best interest then it will probably be advised.

Appropriate first aid measures may be necessary until the patient is transferred to hospital, usually as an emergency. It must be assured that the patient is breathing, that they cannot choke and that they have a pulse.

Overleaf you will find the NICE (National Institute for Health and Clinical Excellence) flow chart ('pathway') which shows in simple way what actions and interventions should be taken at the point of initial assessment of a stroke:

Pathway 1:
Stroke overview

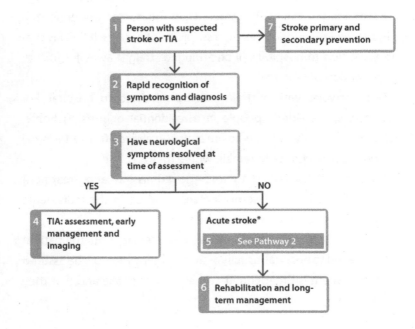

* For Pathway 2, see page 122

National Institute for Health and Clinical Excellence (2008) Adapted from 'Stroke pathway'. London: NICE. Available from www.nice.org.uk. Reproduced with permission.

What happens in hospital

If a stroke is suspected or diagnosed then the sooner the patient is admitted to a hospital stroke unit the better. Not all areas of the country have a stroke unit, in which case the patient may be admitted to the accident and emergency department for the initial assessment, or to an acute medical admissions unit before being transferred to a hospital ward. If a stroke unit is not available, or it is impossible to transfer the patient to one for some reason – perhaps because they are deemed too ill to move – then it is important that they are seen by a specialist with expertise in stroke medicine as soon as possible. This may be a consultant in medicine of the elderly or a consultant neurologist.

In other hospitals, there may be a One-stop Stroke Assessment Unit where a patient will be seen and all the appropriate tests are done as quickly as possible. Some patients may be able to return home under the care of their own doctor, but most patients will be admitted.

What happens next

A full case history will be taken by a doctor, including an account of the event as observed by any witness. The description of what they noticed can be very useful and may fill in gaps that the patient is not aware of. This is particularly valuable if there was loss of consciousness.

The patient's speech, understanding, memory and cooperation will be assessed as the history is taken.

A full physical examination will also be performed, paying particular attention to the neurological examination. Here, the strength and power of all the limbs will be assessed, the reflexes of the upper and lower limbs will be tested and the eyes will be examined, as will most of the cranial nerves. These will give the examining doctor a good idea about which type of stroke it is and which part of the brain has been affected.

Blood pressure will be taken and it will be noted if it is high; the heart will be checked and the neck listened to in order to hear if any bruits are present in the carotid arteries.

Various tests will be repeated over time in order to compare how the symptoms and signs are progressing, either for the better or the worse.

Carotid bruit test

Narrowing of a carotid artery causes turbulence in the flow of blood; its significance is that it indicates some degree of carotid artery disease. When it is present, it may cause carotid artery stenosis, which means significant narrowing of the calibre of the vessel with consequent lessening of supply of blood to the Circle of Willis and, ultimately, to the brain. The doctor listens over the carotid artery with a stethoscope.

CT scan

A Computerised Tomography (CT) scan of the head will be done as soon as possible in order to see whether the cause of the stroke was a haemorrhage. This is essentially a computerised method of assessing a series of X-rays taken at different angles in order to try to build up a series of visual slices of the head. If no blood is seen in the brain then it is probable that the stroke was an ischaemic one.

MRI scan

This is one of the most sophisticated investigations which, if it is available, may be used immediately instead of a CT scan. Unlike the CT scan, it does not use X-rays so no irradiation is involved.

MRI stands for Magnetic Resonance Imaging. It is an investigation which uses magnetism, ultrasound and computerised technology to build up multiple images of the inside of the body. This can show the tissues and any derangement in surprising detail.

It can be an alarming investigation for people who are prone to claustrophobia, since with some scanners it necessitates being advanced through a large tunnel-like apparatus.

Blood tests

A full blood count (FBC) will be done to ascertain the general state of the blood and to check the numbers of the various types of blood cell.

An Erythrocyte Sedimentation Rate (ESR) test will be done to check on the viscosity of the blood and to give an idea about the presence of inflammation, which might lead to a search for conditions like Temporal Arteritis, or Systemic Lupus Erythematosis or other collagen disorders that may predispose to stroke. Blood glucose will be checked to determine whether diabetes is present; if it is already known about, then the check will tell whether or not it is under control. Cholesterol will be checked to see whether levels are high, since this is a risk factor.

Bleeding time may be checked to see if there is a tendency to excessive bleeding.

Other tests may be done as follows:

Chest X-ray

Many patients will be given an X-ray because it will give information about the size of the heart. If the heart is enlarged and the patient has high blood pressure, it indicates whether the heart has been struggling to pump blood through the circulation because of the high pressure. In such circumstances, the heart dilates and becomes less effective as a pump.

ECG

An electrocardiogram (ECG) is a test to determine the electrical activity of the heart. This is useful to see whether there is any abnormal heart rhythm, such as atrial fibrillation; if so, then it is a potential source of a clot or embolism and may have been the underlying reason that the individual had an ischaemic stroke.

It may also give an indication of underlying heart disease, which may also be relevant.

Echocardiogram

This is a non-invasive test that uses sound waves to produce images of the way that the heart is functioning. It can show if there are valve anomalies which could be involved in the production of blood clots or emboli. It is another useful test if there is atrial fibrillation.

Carotid Doppler

This test may be done at some stage. It is a special type of ultrasound examination of the carotid arteries, where a probe is applied over the skin on each side of the neck. It would be indicated if a bruit was heard on the physical examination and is often done in the investigation of someone who has evidence of cerebro-vascular disease, such as a history of repeated TIAs.

Carotid duplex ultrasound

This is a more complex investigation which combines Doppler techniques with ultrasound. It is good at detecting carotid artery stenosis of 50 per cent or greater. A stenosis of 60 per cent in a patient with a history of TIAs may be regarded as a point at which vascular surgery may be advised.

An operation called carotid endarterectomy is used to remove the thickened and narrowed stenosis. However, there is a risk that the procedure itself could cause a stroke and less invasive treatments may be considered first. A stent (small tube) could be placed inside the vessel to keep it open.

Angiogram

Sometimes a stroke team, including a specialist radiologist, may have to perform an angiogram. This is a special type of X-ray that involves dye being injected into a blood vessel in order to highlight a blood vessel that is blocked. It may be possible to then open it up.

What treatment is likely?

This depends upon the very important question of whether the cause has been blockage (ischaemic stroke) or a bleed (haemorrhagic stroke). It is important that this question is answered as quickly as possible, since the longer the brain is deprived of oxygen and essential nutrients, the more brain cells will die off.

No, there is no haemorrhage

This indicates an ischaemic stroke and attempts may need to be made to disperse the clot and to prevent further clotting.

Thrombolytic treatment

Clot-busting or thrombolytic treatment is available for ischaemic strokes. It cannot be given to a patient with haemorrhagic stroke, since it could make the haemorrhage worse.

The thrombolytic drug (and we shall look at them in closer detail in **Chapter 7, Medication**) is given by injection into a vein. It will effectively begin the breakdown of a clot and should help to restore the circulation. It needs to be given as soon as possible after the stroke, within three hours and no longer than four-and-a-half hours.

This is not a treatment that everyone will be offered, since all complex treatments have to be carefully balanced in terms of risk against benefit. The main risk of this drug is that it could cause a haemorrhage in an ischaemic stroke. Perhaps 10–15 per cent of cases will actually receive thrombolytic treatment.

Aspirin or anticoagulants

In addition to the above, either aspirin or an anticoagulant drug should be given as soon as possible. The choice of drug depends upon the clinical picture.

There have been numerous trials on aspirin and its place in the treatment of stroke, and it certainly has a place to offer protection against another stroke. The Royal College of Physicians and NICE currently recommend that patients should be given 300 mg of aspirin after a stroke, as soon as a haemorrhagic stroke has been excluded. In addition, patients should be prescribed 50–300 mg aspirin daily indefinitely.

Patients who have had a mini-stroke should take aspirin, probably 75 mg daily, indefinitely.

If atrial fibrillation is present, then NICE has recommendations about which patients should have aspirin and which should have an anticoagulant, such as warfarin.

The $CHADS_2$ algorithm is used to calculate the risk of having a stroke for patients with non-valvular atrial fibrillation (atrial fibrillation that is not caused by a heart valve problem). It is used to determine whether treatment with anticoagulants or antiplatelet drugs like aspirin is needed.

C = Congestive heart failure

H = Hypertension

A = Age of 75 years or over

D = Diabetes mellitus is present

S2 = Prior stroke TIA or thromboembolism history

One point is allotted to each of the parameters if it is present as above. The greater the $CHADS_2$ score, the greater the risk of stroke within the next year; the lower it is, then the lower the risk.

In addition to indicating risk, $CHADS_2$ gives the recommendation of whether to treat with antiplatelet drugs like aspirin or anticoagulants like warfarin. Since 2012, NICE has recommended that rivaroxaban and dabigatran, two newer anticoagulants, can be used as alternatives to warfarin.

CHADS$_2$ score	Stroke risk %	Recommendation
0	1.9	Aspirin
1	2.8	Aspirin or warfarin
2	4.0	Warfarin
3	5.9	Warfarin
4	8.5	Warfarin
5	12.5	Warfarin
6	18.2	Warfarin

A modified version is also used with additional criteria, which gives more accurate results for lower-risk patients. But for our purposes, the CHADS$_2$ gives the idea.

Thus, in patients with atrial fibrillation classified at low risk of a stroke, with a CHADS$_2$ of zero, a daily dose aspirin of 75 mg to 300 mg should be given, assuming no contraindications.

In patients with atrial fibrillation classified at moderate risk of a stroke, a CHADS$_2$ of 1, a daily dose of 75 mg to 300 mg of aspirin should be given or anticoagulation should be considered.

In patients with atrial fibrillation classified at high risk of a stroke, with a CHADS$_2$ of 2 or above, warfarin should be given to maintain blood-controlled anticoagulation, provided there is no contraindication. If there is a contraindication, then aspirin should be considered, provided there are no contraindications to it.

As noted above since 2012, NICE has recommended that rivaroxaban and dabigatran, two newer anticoagulants, can be used as alternatives to warfarin.

Warfarin is probably 80 per cent likely to prevent clot formation, whereas aspirin is about 20 per cent likely to prevent clots. One would have thought that it would be better to opt for the higher protection, but in medicine it is always a case of balancing risk against benefit. The problems with using warfarin is that there is a significant risk of haemorrhage. In someone who had a large ischaemic area of infarction, there would be a risk of a haemorrhagic stroke.

In many cases, aspirin would be less likely to cause side effects (although it can cause considerable side effects, as we shall see later in **Chapter 7, Medication**).

Clot retrieval

At some specialist stroke centres procedures are being developed to remove blood clots in brain arteries using clot retrieval devices. These are highly sophisticated miniature tools on the ends of very fine catheters, which are inserted into an artery through an incision in the groin. A neuroradiologist, guides the catheter to the site of the clot, using X-ray monitoring. The device then takes hold of the clot and draws it back into the catheter and then removes it from the body.

There are several ways that this can be done. One technique involves a wire being passed through the clot to produce a coil on the far side of it, which then allows the clot to be drawn into the catheter. Another method is to use a tiny wire cage instead of a coil, which enmeshes the clot before removal. Another method uses a vacuum-like device to sucks the clot into the catheter.

These are potentially highly valuable techniques, but they are only available in a small number of centres and much research is still needed on them.

Yes, there has been a haemorrhage

If a haemorrhage has been confirmed then the patient must not have thrombolytic therapy, aspirin or anticoagulants. Their management depends on ascertaining how big the bleed has been, where it has originated from and whether there are any underlying factors or conditions that have caused the bleed. The treatment of those conditions is important and various drugs may need to be taken to get the condition under control. This can be the case in hypertension, various blood disorders or diabetes.

If the haemorrhage has been the result of being on an anticoagulant, then the anticoagulant will be stopped straight away and a drug that counters the effect will be administered intravenously. This could either be a drug called recombinant-activated Factor VII, known as rFVII, which is a blood-clotting factor, or it could be Vitamin K, which counteracts the effect of warfarin.

Surgery

The role of surgery in the acute phase of a stroke has been investigated in several trials. It has not been found to be a prime treatment method, although there are certain indications when it may be necessary, such as:

- With a worsening state in a stroke in a young patient under the age of 60 years

- When a large haematoma or collection of clotted blood may need to be evacuated

- If there is considerable swelling of the brain, to try to relieve the pressure

- If there is cerebellar haemorrhage.

PART 2

DEALING WITH STROKE

An important note about brain plasticity

Before we start looking at recovery and rehabilitation after a stroke, let us consider the important topic of brain plasticity or neuroplasticity.

In a stroke, if brain cells are deprived of blood and oxygen for a critical few minutes, they will die. They will not regenerate. This does not mean that all is lost, because the brain does have the capability of regaining knowledge of or relearning how to do tasks that were dependent upon the part of the brain that has been lost. This capacity is referred to as brain plasticity or neuroplasticity – the ability for the brain to be 'remoulded' into learning new processes, achieved with the help of rehabilitative therapy. Essentially, the work carried out by the patient and the various therapists involved in rehabilitation does somehow stimulate the brain to find new and alternate pathways.

The message is that, even if disabilities are severe and are taking a long time to improve, the brain will be trying its best to find these alternate brain cells and nerve pathways. It will be trying to 'defrag', to use a computer term, and sort out a means of re-routing information and impulses. So, even if a disability seems to be permanent, it may still be possible for the brain to relearn how to do things. The truth is that we still don't understand very much about the way that the brain functions and organises things. Rehabilitation after a stroke is an ongoing process which aims to help exploit the plasticity of the brain to achieve the best outcome.

Mirror-box therapy

There have been several studies which show that the rehabilitation of stroke patients can be improved when physical treatments are combined with mental exercises. It seems that this combination works because of brain plasticity.

The use of a mirror box is something that I would personally recommend. Essentially, it involves using a mirror to create an illusion, tricking the brain into thinking that it is moving a paralysed hand or leg, and so can stimulate improvement. It seems to help the brain to find the alternate route to transmit signals.

Effectively, the patient places the affected limb inside a mirror box and looks at their other limb in the mirror. When they move the normal limb and try to move the paralysed one at the same time, the reflection will give the illusion that they are moving the paralysed limb. The movement may be quite simple, like closing and opening a fist.

This sort of exercise can help. The main thing is to keep practising and keep working with your therapist to achieve results.

Chapter 6

Stroke recovery and rehabilitation

The first few days after a stroke are crucially important; the patient has to be helped to recover as much as possible. In the last chapter, we looked at the investigations that need to be done and the potential use of clot-busting drugs, or aspirin or anticoagulants in the case of ischaemic strokes, in order to prevent further ischaemic strokes from occurring. In this chapter, we take a look at what can be expected in terms of care in the first few days.

Remember that, in those first few days, the stroke may be resolving or the area of the brain affected may still be undergoing changes, as more brain cells may be dying off. It is important that the patient is observed so that any intervention that may be needed is made.

It is, understandably, an intensely frightening experience for someone to find that they have lost the use of part of their body. They need emotional as well as physical support. It is also a troubling time for members of the family so it is useful to know what can be expected in those first days in hospital. The stroke team will support the patient and keep them informed about how they are progressing.

How long in hospital?

This varies according to the type and severity of the stroke, but almost half of all patients who have a stroke will make a full or near-full recovery within a week. They are considered to have had either a TIA, if they have recovery from all symptoms and signs within 24 hours, or a mild stroke if it resolves in a few more days up to a week.

Those for whom the symptoms and signs last longer than a week are generally regarded as having had a moderate or a severe stroke. They will require longer rehabilitation before they can be discharged home to live independently. Others may not recover enough for that to happen and they may have to be admitted to a nursing home or a residential home.

KEY POINTS

- Patients admitted to a stroke unit make a better recovery than those admitted to a general ward.
- Symptoms present in the first few days may very well disappear.
- If symptoms are going to improve they will usually do so within two months.
- Symptoms lasting six months are liable to be permanent.

The stroke unit

As mentioned earlier, the ideal situation is for a patient to be admitted to a specialised stroke unit where they can be assessed and looked after by a team of professionals specifically trained in the care of the patient with a stroke.

There is good evidence from the 2007 Stroke Unit Trialists' Collaboration study of 31 trials, involving 6,939 participants, that patients do better in stroke units than in general hospital wards.[4] In particular, they found that people admitted to a stroke unit were more likely to be alive, independent and living at home one year later. They also found that, after five years and ten years, people who had been treated in a stroke unit were more likely to be living at home and be less disabled.

Another meta-analysis found that any type of specialist stroke care worked better than non-specialist care.[5] This makes it clear that it is preferable to be treated in a stroke unit, where the trained staff only treat people with strokes.

The three types of stroke unit

Acute or intensive stroke units – are where the immediate treatment of the stroke patient takes place. They are admitted directly to the unit and given all appropriate tests and treatment.

Rehabilitation stroke units – are where the patient is admitted after seven days from the stroke. The focus here is not on the acute episode, but on helping the patient back to health and restoring as much function as possible.

Combined acute and rehabilitation units – are where a patient is admitted as soon as they have had a stroke and where they will receive rehabilitation for several weeks.

The problems that need to be dealt with

The care of a patient with a stroke necessitates teamwork. Different members of the team will bring different areas of expertise. In particular, the following potential problems may need to be focused upon.

Consciousness

This is, of course, fundamental. A patient may become comatose after a stroke and their level of consciousness will be assessed using a scoring system that depends on concrete measurable parameters. Their level of consciousness needs to be monitored closely in order to assess improvement or deterioration. This is of importance as it affects whatever intervention will be needed.

Swallowing difficulty

If the part of the brain that controls the swallowing mechanism is damaged during a stroke, then the person's ability to swallow may be affected. This is vitally important because the airway and the oesophagus (the tube which carries food and drink down the stomach) both have the same opening at the back of the throat. If the swallowing mechanism is not present, then food or drink could go into the lungs rather than the stomach. This could either obstruct the airway and cause death very quickly from asphyxiation, or produce an aspiration pneumonia, which could also be fatal.

One of the first things that is performed on a conscious stroke patient is a swallowing test. This assesses the individual's ability to swallow a sample of water, and is carried out by either the nursing staff or a speech therapist.

No stroke patient should be given food, drink or medication until this test has been done.

Hydration and nutrition problems

If anyone is unable to take food or drink because of their stroke, they may be fitted with a nasogastric tube through which they can be given food and fluids. This should be done within 24 hours of admission. Some people can get quite dehydrated after a stroke and they may require an intravenous drip to be set up so that fluids can be administered directly into the circulation through a vein. Drugs can also be given by this route.

The state of hydration will be monitored clinically, and possibly also by blood tests to measure plasma osmolality (the body's electrolyte–water balance). If a patient is unable to tolerate a nasogastric tube, then a PEG tube may be inserted directly through the stomach and out through the abdominal wall. PEG stands for Percutaneous Endoscopically-placed Gastroenterostomy tube, since the technique is done by performing an endoscopy, which involves a trained person passing a fibre-optic endoscope into the stomach. The PEG is then positioned so that the tube leads directly into the stomach. It is a simple technique that takes about 20 minutes and requires only mild sedation and local anaesthetic. A PEG tube may have to be used for a long time and some patients may have to use it permanently.

Support for the body's homoeostasis

Homoeostasis means the body's ability to self-regulate its internal environment. This ability can be affected in stroke patients in the early stages and particular care needs to be taken by the medical and nursing staff to monitor several parameters. It has been shown that when blood pressure, oxygen saturation, temperature and blood sugar levels are analysed and maintained that the outcome of stroke is improved.

Oxygen saturation is a measure of the oxygen that is being carried by your red blood cells. Normally 95–100 per cent of them are loaded with oxygen, hence 'saturation'. This can be measured by a light sensor clipped to a finger. If it is less than 95 per cent saturation, then oxygen can be given by a mask.

Blood glucose should be maintained between the levels of 4 and 11 mmol/litre. Blood pressure should also be monitored. This is certainly something that will need to be looked at later, so there may not be much alteration of treatment or initiation of treatment, unless there is evidence of hypertensive damage to the brain, kidneys, heart or evidence of a haemorrhagic stroke with a systolic pressure of greater than 200 mmHg. Treatment would also be considered for people who are about to receive thrombolytic treatment and who have a blood pressure reading of greater than 185/110. Temperature needs to be monitored, since a raised temperature could indicate an infection somewhere that needs treatment.

Paralysed limbs

Special care has to be taken of paralysed limbs to prevent injury. The shoulder joints in particular are vulnerable and it is important that they are positioned correctly and moved appropriately and carefully. The physiotherapist is of inestimable value here, assessing each case individually.

KEY POINTS

- The majority of stroke patients regain the ability to walk.
- 85 per cent of stroke patients have upper limb impairments after a stroke.
- 30–60 per cent recover the use of the upper limb affected to a functional level.
- Only 15 per cent regain hand function.[6]

Prevention of spasticity

Spasticity is a state in which skeletal muscles can change to become tight, stiff and even rigid. It can easily occur in a paralysed limb and it should be prevented if possible. If spasticity of a limb occurs then treatment should be initiated with various physiotherapy techniques and possibly also with various drugs. It is quite important to do all that is possible to maintain the strength of muscles that are affected by spasticity.

In patients with disabling or symptomatically distressing spasticity, injection of botulinum toxin should be considered in conjunction with physiotherapy for reducing tone and/or increasing the range of joint motion. Sometimes, electro-stimulation should also be considered to increase the effectiveness of the botulinum toxin.

Continence of bowels and bladder

This is of vital importance. In the past, patients with stroke often used to be catheterised to prevent incontinence of urine. Nowadays, catheterisation is to be prevented as much as possible.

Very often a stroke patient is distressed or embarrassed by having an accident and involuntarily passing faeces or urine. This will be handled sensitively by the stroke team and the individual will be given all help needed to gain independence. For some time, however, they may need help with incontinence pads, bottles, bedpans or commodes.

Many units have a continence advisor who is specially trained in dealing and advising with all problems of continence of bowels and bladder. Bowel function may be disturbed and either constipation or looseness of motions may develop. The nursing staff are quite expert in juggling diet, fluids and laxatives if necessary to maintain continence. Catheterisation is used only when absolutely necessary.

Early mobilisation

One of the prime aims is to mobilise the patient as soon as possible. It is not good to lie for too long, since there is increased risk of venous thrombosis, bedsores and muscle wasting. As we shall see later, the physiotherapist and nursing staff will try to help the individual to sit as soon as possible. Walking will be a priority, as soon as it is considered reasonable and possible by the therapist.

The stroke team and who does what

The stroke team will consist of:

- Medical staff

- Nursing staff

- Speech therapist

- Physiotherapist

- Occupational therapist

- Psychologist

- Social worker

- Pharmacist

- Dietician

- Ophthalmologist and orthoptist.

Medical staff

The team will consist of a consultant who will take overall responsibility for the patient's medical care. This will possibly be a consultant in stroke medicine or a consultant in care of the elderly, or a consultant neurologist. He/she will be supported by a team of junior doctors.

The medical staff will do the physical examinations and arrange whatever tests are needed in order to accurately diagnose the type of stroke the patient has had and assess its severity. If the patient is comatose then they will arrange care of breathing, monitor level of consciousness and ensure that patient is properly hydrated. This will necessitate putting up an intravenous infusion, commonly called a drip, that will replace fluids directly into a vein.

All blood tests to monitor the function of the liver and kidneys will be arranged by the doctors. Blood samples may be taken by the doctors or by specially trained phlebotomists (technicians trained in putting up intravenous drips and taking blood for testing). They will also monitor oxygen levels. If the oxygen saturation falls below 95 per cent then oxygen may be given.

The doctors will prescribe any medication that needs to be given.

Nursing staff

The nursing staff will be the members that the patient has most to do with. They will tend to the patient's daily needs and will help with their dressing, washing, going to the toilet and eating and drinking. They will ensure that the patient is as comfortable as possible and is not in a position where they can injure any joints.

They are experts on preventing bedsores and in ensuring that bowel and bladder support is given. They will also keep the patient's limbs moving to reduce the risk of a deep vein thrombosis developing in a paralysed limb.

Nursing staff are also concerned with helping the patient to mobilise and they will continue the care that is given by other professionals. If oxygen is needed, they will administer it.

Speech therapist

These professionals have an essential role in stroke rehabilitation. A speech therapist is likely to see the patient soon after admission, in order to do a swallowing assessment. This is vital, since a stroke patient must not be given any food or drink until it has been ascertained whether or not they have an intact swallowing mechanism. If not, then it would be dangerous for them to be given food or drink that could be aspirated into the lungs.

The speech therapist also will make an assessment of the patient's ability to understand and communicate. If there are any speech problems, then they will start to work on them with the patient and the other staff.

If a patient has significant aphasia problems, the therapist will do a lot of work with symbols and pictures in order to help the patient relearn words and sentences.

Variants of aphasia

Expressive aphasia – when the individual knows what they want to say or write, but has difficulty with speech. This arises when Broca's area is affected (see Chapter 1) and it is sometimes known as Broca's aphasia.

Receptive aphasia – when the individual can hear the voice of another person, but cannot interpret or understand it. Their speech may retain its fluency, but some of the words may be nonsensical and sentences may have mistakes in them. This arises when Wernicke's area is affected (see Chapter 1) and it is sometimes known as Wernicke's aphasia.

Anomic aphasia – when the individual has difficulty in finding words or names. Many people have this problem, called anomia, but a stroke may make it worse and more distressing.

Global aphasia – this occurs when both speech and the understanding of words are lost. There may also be loss of the ability to read and write. It is usually as result of a larger stroke affecting both Broca's and Wernicke's areas.

Physiotherapist

The physiotherapist is a vital member of the team. The recommendation is that there should be the equivalent of one or two full-time staff per ten-bed stroke unit.

The aim in the stroke unit is to mobilise the person as soon as possible. This is essential, since the longer one is immobile the more chance there is of spasticity developing. This can be a huge problem for a stroke survivor and it is to be avoided at all costs.

The physiotherapist will make their initial assessment of the patient's posture, their ability to sit, stand and walk. If the patient cannot sit without support then they will give advice on the best way to position limbs in order to prevent injury.

It is also very important to get the patient sitting as soon as possible to minimise the risk of complications such as aspiration of fluids into the lungs, respiratory complications, shoulder pain, contractures and pressure sores. All of those are potential problems if the patient is bed-bound.

Shoulder problems are a particular problem after stroke as this area can become very stiff. In order to prevent shoulder pain, overhead arm slings should be avoided, since these encourage uncontrolled abduction (forcing the arm and shoulder upwards). A physiotherapist will also advise on the use of foam supports and other aids and hoists if they are required.

The regime of exercises to be used will be very much tailored to the needs of the patient. Goals should be organised and agreed with the patient so that they are actively involved in their own rehabilitation, and are not just a recipient of physiotherapy treatment.

Every patient who has had a stroke is keen to walk as soon as they can. The stroke team may try to delay this until the physiotherapist is sure that they are ready to do so. Mobilisation is extremely important, but it has to be managed well. Walking may have to be relearned and it is of prime importance that falls should be avoided and also that bad walking habits are not developed.

Walking aids, ranging from Zimmer frames to walking sticks, may be needed and the physiotherapist will advise accordingly. Indeed, this area is very important since the walking aid needs to be right for the person and their individual needs.

The patient and their family or potential carers will also be involved, so that they have an understanding of how they can continue to help the stroke survivor to improve.

At some stage, the patient may receive some of their treatment in a special gym in order to relearn how to walk or to help improve posture, gait and strength.

Occupational therapist

The role of this therapist is to help the stroke survivor to assess and manage the tasks of daily life, usually referred to as the activities of daily living. These include the individual's ability to wash, bathe or shower, feed themselves and go to the toilet.

As the rehabilitation progresses, they also assess the extended activities of daily living, including cooking, shopping, managing hobby or leisure activities, driving and using public transport.

The occupational therapist will advise on the use of various types of aids, such as:

- Gripping and turning aids

- Kettle and teapot tippers

- Kitchen aids

- Large-handled cutlery

- Reachers and grabbing gadgets

- Special drinking cups and mugs

- Walking trolleys.

The occupational therapist will probably be involved later on in the health and social care assessment. This may be done during a home visit if the patient is sufficiently recovered for discharge to home.

Psychologist

While most people recover well after a stroke, some may develop psychological problems which can impede their recovery. A clinical psychologist can assess any difficulties that the patient is experiencing with their thinking and understanding. They may then decide what type of psychological treatment will be most beneficial.

Social worker

The social worker may well be asked to help with various matters relating to the stroke survivor's needs. There may be a need to organise various types of social support after discharge and to help the patient with regards to various benefits that they may wish to apply for.

Together with the other professionals, the social worker will be involved in the discharge management plan and may be involved in the discussion and report arising from the health and social care assessment.

Pharmacist

Many stroke survivors find that they are discharged whilst taking several different medications. The pharmacist will liaise with the medical staff to arrange the most appropriate drugs. There may be problems about whether a drug needs to be taken as a solid tablet, a capsule or in suspension, solution or even as a suppository.

The patient will also be discharged home with a supply of the appropriate drugs.

After discharge, the community pharmacist may liaise with the family doctor to arrange ongoing drug supplies, possibly including delivery to the home, if needed, and supplying dosset boxes to help simplify the drug-taking process.

Dosset boxes have different rows of compartments for each day, so that each day's supply is made up with compartments for the different times of the day. Thus, each drug is placed in the appropriate compartment with others that are to be taken at the same time. This enables the user or carer to ensure that the right drugs are taken at the right times.

Dietician

The nutritional status of the individual with a stroke needs great care, especially if they are unable to take food and drink orally. A nasogastric tube or a PEG may solve the immediate problem, but there is a risk with this if there has been a period of starvation beforehand when no nutrients were being given. This can lead to a problem called 're-feeding syndrome'. This was first observed in prisoners of war during World War Two who had suffered from malnutrition – the sudden presence of food can lead to dangerous alteration in mineral and electrolyte levels. All such patients would benefit from close liaison between medical staff and dietician.

Ophthalmologist and orthoptist

Strokes often affect people's vision; this can be minor or very severe. An assessment by an opthalmologist can be very helpful to determine the extent of impairment of vision, which may be followed by a referral to an orthoptist, a therapist trained in dealing with eye exercises and the use of various optical aids.

Pathways of care

One of the main advantages in having a specialised stroke unit is that all aspects of stroke care will be considered and addressed. Many stroke units will have a pathway of care map that is used to organise the ways and the times so that the patient gets all the tests and treatments that they should receive. The patient is likely to receive a detailed but comprehensible plan of what will happen each day. This ensures that the patient will receive the best standard of care and that nothing is missed.

NICE, the National Institute for Health and Clinical Excellence, has created a whole range of these flow charts, or pathways, which show in simple ways what actions and interventions should be taken at various stages of a case.

Pathway 2:
Acute stroke

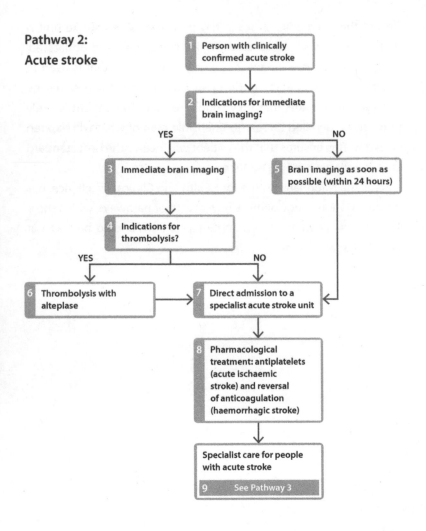

1. Person with clinically confirmed acute stroke

2. Indications for immediate brain imaging?

   YES → 3. Immediate brain imaging

   NO → 5. Brain imaging as soon as possible (within 24 hours)

4. Indications for thrombolysis?

   YES → 6. Thrombolysis with alteplase

   NO → 7. Direct admission to a specialist acute stroke unit

7. Direct admission to a specialist acute stroke unit

8. Pharmacological treatment: antiplatelets (acute ischaemic stroke) and reversal of anticoagulation (haemorrhagic stroke)

Specialist care for people with acute stroke

9. See Pathway 3

Pathway 3:

Specialist care for people with acute stroke

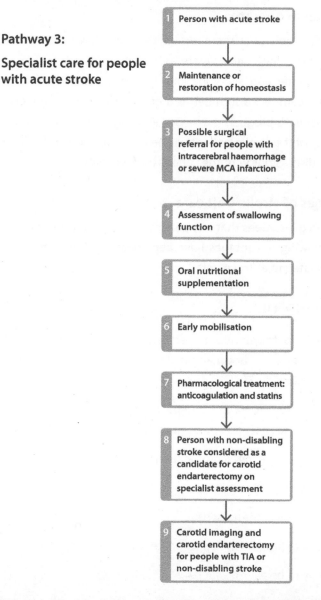

1. Person with acute stroke

2. Maintenance or restoration of homeostasis

3. Possible surgical referral for people with intracerebral haemorrhage or severe MCA infarction

4. Assessment of swallowing function

5. Oral nutritional supplementation

6. Early mobilisation

7. Pharmacological treatment: anticoagulation and statins

8. Person with non-disabling stroke considered as a candidate for carotid endarterectomy on specialist assessment

9. Carotid imaging and carotid endarterectomy for people with TIA or non-disabling stroke

National Institute for Health and Clinical Excellence (2008) Adapted from 'Stroke pathway'. London: NICE. Available from www.nice.org.uk. Reproduced with permission.

How the team operates

Although the individual members of the team have their areas of responsibility, they will operate as a team so that the care all dovetails together and everyone knows what is being done for a patient. The team will also meet as a group at least once a week, when the patient's progress is assessed and ongoing care planned.

The family of the stroke patient will be kept informed and will be involved in discussions with the various professionals.

Advantages of stroke unit care

There are no guarantees that any patient will recover from a stroke, but the following advantages have been demonstrated when the patient is treated in a stroke unit.

The stroke survivor is:

- More likely to be monitored regularly over the first 48 hours, rather than on an ad hoc manner as it can be fitted in to a general ward's working

- Less likely to have complications, due to better monitoring of heart rate, oxygen levels and temperature

- Less likely to get respiratory infections

- Less likely to get urinary infections

- Less likely to be catheterised

- More likely to have all the appropriate tests

- More likely to be alive a year later

- Less likely to be disabled

- More likely to be able to live independently

- More likely to be able to live at home one year after a stroke

- More likely to be discharged from hospital sooner. It has been found that stroke unit patients are discharged between two and six days sooner than stroke patients treated in a general ward

- Less likely to be readmitted.

In addition, and very importantly, it does not matter what type of stroke the patient has had, or how old they are or how severe the stroke was – the stroke unit seems to offer the best care and the best outcome. NICE recommends that all patients should be offered admission to a specialist acute stroke clinic.

The Health and Social Care Assessment

Rehabilitation may take several weeks or even months in hospital, and the aim is to get the patient to the best possible state of health before they can be discharged from the unit. The majority of patients will be able to return to their home, but others may require alternative arrangements, either in a residential home or in a nursing home. This really reflects the level of functional independence that is obtained.

When a patient is considered ready to be discharged from hospital, then the local authority will carry out a Health and Social Care Assessment. This is usually done by an occupational therapist, who will assess an individual's physical, psychological, social and cultural needs. This may involve a visit to the home with the patient and the carer or other members of the family. The therapist will assess how suitable the home is in terms of whether aids and adaptations need to be installed – e.g. bath rails, toilet raises, handrails, stair lifts and ramps – and they will assess it from the point of view of the carer as well as the stroke patient. They will also assess how well the patient can manage on their own or with the help of their carer.

This will all be discussed at another team meeting prior to actual discharge. The point is that the patient and carer must feel happy and confident that they are going to be able to cope, so this joint visit will be therapeutic as well as having a practical function.

It may be necessary to arrange a package of care, involving the visits of social carers, nurses and the family doctor. Liaison is important so that there is a neat transition from hospital care to community care. A report will be made and the person with the stroke will be given a copy.

The following services may be arranged with the help of social services:

- Advice about finance and any benefits that may be appropriate

- Equipment and aids to help with daily living

- Arrangements for attendance at day centres

- Home help or care assistant visits

- Meals on wheels

- Respite care in residential or nursing home or short stay in hospital (this may be important for any carers)

- Permanent residential or nursing home care.

KEY POINTS

- About 60 per cent of stroke patients will return home and be able to live independently.
- About 15 per cent will be able to live at home with a carer or a care package.

We shall look at alterations that may need to be made to the home in a little more detail in **Chapter 10, Life after a stroke.**

Care homes

If a person's disability is such that they will be unable to live independently at home, then it may be recommended that they move into a care home, which vary in the facilities that they offer. Until recently, care homes were classified as being either residential or a nursing home – now the differentiation is according to whether they provide 'personal care and nursing care'.

Moving into a care home can be an alarming prospect, since it may be a radical change of life. It also will have financial implications and a financial assessment will need to be done by the local authority and social services to see what proportion the person will have to fund themselves.

All care homes are regulated by official bodies:

The Care Quality Commission (CQC) in England

The Care and Social Services Inspectorate in Wales (CSSIW)

The Scottish Commission for the Regulation of Care in Scotland (SCRC)

The Regulation and Quality Improvement Authority in Northern Ireland (RQIA)

Residential care homes

Here, a person will have their own room, usually with en-suite facilities, and the use of a communal sitting room and dining room. Support will be available 24 hours a day. These are mainly for people who need some support, but who have no major nursing needs.

Such care homes are run by various organisations – they may be local authority homes, private companies or voluntary organisations. A choice will be available and social services will be able to provide a list of care homes in the patient's local area. It is a big decision as to which one will be best, and it is advisable to ask the family to visit and ascertain as much information as possible about the home. This includes finding out about facilities, type of food available and what sort of social amenities the home provides. It is a decision about where the person is going to live and they need to feel comfortable about it.

Nursing homes (care home providing personal care and nursing care)

These are homes where nursing input is available to help people with more significant disabilities and medical conditions. Trained nursing staff will be assisted by care assistants.

This is the place that is likely to be needed if a person requires access to a nurse at any time during the day. This would relate to people needing care in bed, or if there is a medical problem requiring regular nursing or medical care.

Funding your stay in a care home

It is likely that a patient's stay in a care home will have to be funded privately, i.e. paid for by the patient or a family member. How much private funding is required will vary according to which country you live in; your local authority can carry out a financial assessment, undertaken by a social worker. They will consider the patient's circumstances, including the following areas:

- Income (including pensions)

- Savings

- Assets

- Benefits

- Outgoings, e.g. mortgage, rent, insurance fees.

One of the things that people worry about is whether the family home will have to be sold to finance a care home. It may be that it will, if the individual had been previously living on their own and then have to go into a care home permanently, and if, after all of the above income and expenditure have been taken into account in the financial assessment, they are still required to make a contribution.

The home will not be taken into account if:

- A spouse or civil partner or a relative who is 60 or over continues to live in the home.

- A disabled or incapacitated relative aged under 60 continues to live in the home.

- A child under 16 years continues to live in the home.

Sheltered accommodation

Yet another option is sheltered accommodation, suitable for the individual who is still able to live independently yet does not feel secure enough to live on their own in their own home.

Again, a number of organisations, including local authority, voluntary organisations and housing associations, operate these. Housing associations may rent out the accommodation or it can be bought as a property.

Sheltered accommodation usually takes the form of a block of small flats, each with a bedroom, toilet, sitting room and a kitchen. A warden or manager will be on hand to manage the scheme and to advise on local services, and perhaps to liaise with services in an emergency. Their remits vary and it is imperative to know and understand how much, if any, assistance they can offer an individual. They do not offer personal care and are often more involved in the bricks and mortar of the building rather than the medical and social care of the residents.

Chapter 7

Medication

When a stroke occurs one can go from being someone who takes no medication to someone who takes many different types of drug. This can be confusing, so we will look at drugs that may be prescribed, when and why.

Drugs that may be prescribed in the initial treatment

These drugs are not suitable for everyone, as should be clear from the previous chapters, since some strokes are ischaemic, due to blockage of arteries, and others are haemorrhagic, due to blood vessels rupturing. Accurate diagnosis is essential and must be backed up by brain imaging in order to be precise.

Clot-busters – thrombolytic drugs

Thanks to the beneficial effects that have been shown by the use of thrombolytic drugs in patients after a myocardial infarction (heart attack), thrombolytic drugs, otherwise known as clot-busters, may be indicated in people with a proven ischaemic stroke, in whom an intracranial haemorrhage has been excluded.

The drug alteplase is given intravenously, but it is only given in special units where the staff are fully trained in administering it and in monitoring for any complications. There must be a facility to have immediate brain-imaging, and re-imaging if necessary, to ensure that a haemorrhage does not occur as a result.

There is a narrow window of opportunity with this drug. It should be given within three hours of the onset of a stroke, after a haemorrhage has been excluded.

Since haemorrhage is a possible side effect, NICE suggests that, if a patient has very high blood pressure, it may be necessary to administer blood-pressure-lowering drugs to bring the pressure down to 185/110 or lower in patients who are candidates for thrombolysis.

Aspirin and antiplatelet drugs

Aspirin is antithrombotic – this means that it prevents the formation of thrombus, or blood clot. It is also called an antiplatelet drug, because it stops platelets from sticking together and producing a blood clot.

Aspirin is known to have many beneficial effects. It is a painkiller, an anti-pyretic (lowers temperature) and an anti-inflammatory drug. More and more research is demonstrating that in low daily doses it reduces the risk of heart attacks, strokes and various types of cancer. Its effectiveness arises because it blocks the action of two cyclo-oxygenase enzymes, known as COX-1 and COX-2. Both are involved in complex metabolic pathways that produce natural chemicals called prostaglandins.

COX-1 has a protective effect on the stomach and is also present in the platelets, the very smallest blood cells that clump together and help to produce a clot. This clumping of platelets is generally a beneficial effect in the body, because it is the way that we heal wounds. On the other hand, when it produces a clot inside a blood vessel, it is extremely dangerous.

COX-2 is involved in the production of specific prostaglandins which start the inflammatory process.

NICE recommends that 300 mg of aspirin should be given as soon as possible to patients with an ischaemic stroke, and certainly within the first 24 hours. It should not be given to anyone who is allergic to it, if they have previously had a haemorrhagic tendency or if they have had a dyspepsia problem with it.

It should be continued for two weeks or until the patient is discharged from hospital if that is sooner. Then they should have long-term antithrombotic treatment with aspirin or with another antithrombotic drug such as dipyridamole or clopidogrel or ticlopidine.

It may be necessary in some patients with past mild dyspepsia to give a proton-pump inhibitor drug such as omeprazole at the same time.

The dosage of aspirin needed to prevent a second stroke is usually 75 mg to 150 mg.

Aspirin has lots of potential side effects. You should never take aspirin if you:

- Have had a haemorrhagic stroke

- Have a history of stomach ulceration

- Have a history of asthma

- Have any blood disorder or inherited condition, which could predispose you to bleeding

- Have had an allergic reaction to aspirin at any time in your life. There would be the danger of having an anaphylactic reaction, which is a serious, potentially life-threatening allergic reaction characterised by low blood pressure, shock and difficulty breathing. It is a medical emergency

- Are under 16 years old

- Are on drugs like anticoagulants, or other drugs which could interact with aspirin to increase the risk of a bleed.

Anticoagulants

These drugs effectively thin the blood and prevent the blood from coagulating (forming a clot). They may be used in patients who have had a venous sinus thrombosis, one of the rarer forms of stroke, which we looked at in **Chapter 2, What happens in a stroke**.

Generally, their role is in the treatment of underlying conditions which may predispose the individual to clot formation, such as atrial fibrillation.

Warfarin has been the main oral anticoagulant up until recently. It necessitates having a regular blood test called an INR (International Normalised Ratio) every two weeks to monitor the level of anticoagulation that has been achieved. The daily dosage can then be varied according to the local anticoagulant clinic whose staff will do the monitoring.

More recently, NICE has approved two other oral anticoagulants – dabigatran and rivaroxaban – in the treatment of patients with atrial fibrillation, in order to reduce their risk of stroke. They both work in different ways from warfarin, but they have the advantage in not having to have regular monitoring and dose adjustment. NICE recommends that these two can be used in patients with non-valvular atrial fibrillation, meaning atrial fibrillation in the absence of a heart valve problem. For patients with atrial fibrillation and a known heart valve problem, warfarin is still the drug of choice.

Cholesterol-lowering drugs

For patients with raised cholesterol levels, a statin drug may be offered, as well as advice on how to lower their cholesterol through dietary means.

NICE does not recommend that statins are started immediately after an acute stroke, but the consensus of opinion of the Guideline Development Group is that it is safe to start them after 48 hours from the onset of the stroke.

The statins, or HMG-CoA reductase inhibitors, have been used for several years to reduce cholesterol levels. They work by inhibiting the enzyme HMG-CoA reductase, which is involved in cholesterol synthesis. The statins work to reduce the level of the enzyme in the liver, which will result in a decrease in the level of cholesterol. They also increase the synthesis of LDL receptors, which helps them to clear low-density lipoproteins from the blood.

Some people react to statins, developing muscle cramps and an inflammatory condition of the muscles called a myopathy. At its extreme form, myopathy can cause a breakdown in muscle tissue (rhabdomyolysis). Nerve damage is also a rare possibility.

Yet, having said that, most people tolerate statins and if one statin produces side effects then another in the group may be tolerated well.

Anti-hypertensives

High blood pressure or hypertension is the most common cause of stroke, as discussed in **Chapter 4, Risk factors for having a stroke and how to reduce your risk**. It is a condition that can creep up on one insidiously, so it is sensible for all adults to have regular blood-pressure checks. For many people who suffer a stroke it may come as a surprise that their blood pressure has been found to be raised. Lowering the blood pressure to an acceptable level is of paramount importance and the process will be started in the hospital and be continued and monitored in general practice.

There are several different types of anti-hypertensive drugs and there are recommended prescribing regimes from NICE. The choice of drugs, or the combination of drugs, may depend on age, other medical conditions and response to one or more drugs.

The drug groups include:

- Calcium channel blockers

- ACE inhibitor or Angiotensin II receptor blockers

- Thiazide diuretics

- Alpha-blocking drugs

- Beta-blocking drugs.

It may be that a patient needs one, two or three types of anti-hypertensive drug. This may take some getting used to, but they are potentially life-saving.

Diabetes care

Diabetes is one of the main causes of stroke. Once again, many people are not aware that they have the condition until a medical problem such as a stroke arises.

If someone discovers that they have diabetes only when they are admitted to hospital with a stroke then they will have the additional challenge of accepting the nature of diabetes. It is vitally important that they understand how crucial it is to maintain good diabetic control from then on.

Diabetes mellitus is a disorder of carbohydrate metabolism from too little insulin, or from a lack of response to the body's own insulin. The characteristic feature of it in an undiagnosed or untreated form is excessive thirst and increased tendency to pass urine.

As mentioned in **Chapter 4, Risk factors for having a stroke and how to reduce your risk,** there are three types of diabetes mellitus:

Type 1 – insulin-dependent diabetes, IDDM. It is due to a failure to produce insulin. It has to be treated with regular injections of insulin. It usually starts in early adult life.

Type 2 – non-insulin-dependent diabetes mellitus, NIDDM. This is due to lack of response to the body's insulin. Weight control and oral hypoglycaemic drugs may be needed.

Gestational diabetes – which can occur in pregnancy.

If diabetes is present, then it will be taken into account in the $ABCD^2$ score in the initial assessment of stroke, as discussed in **Chapter 5, When a stroke strikes.**

The individual's diabetic control will need to be discussed and advice given on lifestyle and diet. Obviously, if the stroke patient is left with a sensory problem in a lower limb and they are diabetic, then they may need to involve the services of a podiatrist.

Other conditions

Some patients may have had their stroke as the result of other underlying conditions, such as blood disorders or inflammatory conditions. The treatment of those conditions may involve other hospital specialties, such as haematology or rheumatology, and the possibility of having to take other drugs.

Compliance

This is the name given to describe how well patients follow medical advice. In 2003, the World Health Organization estimated that in developed countries only 50 per cent of people with chronic conditions follow the medical recommendations that have been given to them. In particular, people tend not to follow the advice or take the medication prescribed for them in hypertension and diabetes.

For anyone who has had a stroke it is essential to be a good complier with whatever drugs have been prescribed to prevent a second stroke, or to control underlying conditions like hypertension and diabetes.

Chapter 8

Complications after a stroke

Recovery from a stroke can take a variable amount of time and, as we have already discussed, not everyone does make a full recovery. The fact is that a stroke is a serious event and no two people recover in the same way. Other conditions can occur to complicate that recovery; diagnosing them is important, since they are all amenable to treatment.

Depression

Understandably, given the grave nature of a stroke, and the fact that one is a stroke survivor, many people get depressed. The stroke makes one aware of how fragile life is and that the stroke that they have just had could have been fatal.

About one third of stroke survivors become depressed. Men tend to become more depressed than women, although the reason why is as yet unclear. A study published in the *Archives of Physical Medicine and Rehabilitation* in 2012 suggested that it may have something to do with the sense of loss of control over life.[7]

The attitude of people around the patient can be very important in helping to counteract this; again this is where a stroke unit has advantages, since the professionals are more used to dealing with people who have sustained all types of stroke. Because it is a specialised unit, the patient is likely to feel that they are receiving the best care possible and may feel safer as a result.

Depression may make a person feel weepy; they may notice that they are worse in the morning and tend to get less depressed as the day goes on. Apathy is common, so a person may need encouragement to cooperate with their treatment. They may lose their appetite and/or they may complain that there is simply no point in their treatment or in them going on living. These are all indicative of a marked depression.

Positive support is what is needed and many people will respond to this after a few days. For those who do not begin to feel better, it may be necessary for them to have an antidepressant – the choice of which one will be decided by the medical staff. It is likely that an antidepressant will need to be taken for several weeks, and more often than not for several months, when it can then be stopped. They usually do not start working for about a week to two weeks.

KEY POINTS

- Most people feel saddened after a stroke for a few days. That is normal.
- One third of stroke survivors become depressed. Not all will need antidepressant medication.

Emotional change

In addition to feeling depressed there is a whole panoply of other emotions that a stroke survivor may experience. Some people become very angry and bitter, others feel guilty and still others may be subject to mood swings.

In part, this may reflect what is going on in the mind as a result of one's reaction to the knowledge that a stroke has occurred; in part, it may relate to which area of the brain has been affected.

The midbrain or limbic system is the emotional brain. This is considered to be part of the brainstem in clinical medicine (see **Chapter 1, Understand the brain**). Thus, strokes affecting this area may produce more emotional change.

Sometimes, family members may comment that they noticed a change in someone's emotional tendency for some time before the stroke occurred. For example, people can seem to get irritable and develop a shorter fuse before the onset of a stroke.

Case study

A 75-year-old man became more and more bad tempered for about two months prior to having an ischaemic stroke in the vicinity of his limbic system. His wife commented that he seemed to be working up to the point where he just blew a fuse.

It is likely that the gradual process of arteriosclerosis, or hardening of the arteries in that part of the brain, was causing some oxygen depletion, affecting his limbic system.

Personality and behaviour change

This seems to be more likely with strokes affecting the frontal area of the brain. This can be quite dramatic with a definite change in the individual's personality as they recover from the initial stoke. There may be a loss of social awareness with inappropriate behaviour, irritability, intolerance and impulsiveness.

Previously prim and proper individuals may swear, use inappropriate language or lose the sense of social limits. They may lose the need to cover themselves in public.

Sometimes after a stroke people may seem to lose the habit of a lifetime – a heavy drinker may lose the taste for alcohol or a chain-smoker may forget the urge to smoke. These seem to be more common when a part of the brain called the insula is affected.

The insula – the seat of smoking addiction

The insula was first described by Johann Christian Reil, a German physician, anatomist and physiologist in the early nineteenth century. He was actually the very first doctor to use the word 'psychiatry' in 1808. He described the insula as a prune-sized area of matter which is found in each side of the brain. It was called the Island of Reil after him, but exactly what its function was he had no way of knowing.

A paper published in the journal *Science* in 2007 was inspired by a patient who smoked 40 cigarettes a day before having a stroke that damaged his insula.[8] He stopped smoking immediately, telling doctors that he 'forgot the urge to smoke'. The scientists then turned to a database of stroke patients held by the University of Iowa and identified 69 people who had smoked at least five cigarettes a day for at least two years before they suffered brain damage. They found that 19 of these patients had damage to the insula and 13 of them had given up smoking, 12 of them quickly and easily. The other six continued to smoke – possibly reflecting damage to different parts of the insula.

It seems that the insula is a complex sort of receiving zone within the brain. It monitors the physiological state of the whole body and then generates feelings that can bring about actions which maintain a state of internal balance. Information from the insula seems to be sent on to higher-functioning areas within the brain in the prefrontal cortex, which are involved in decision-making.

In the smoking scenario above, it seems that the insula becomes accustomed to a blood level of nicotine. If that level drops, the insula is stimulated and sends messages to the higher parts of the brain that perceive a need to get the nicotine level back up, so the person reaches for a cigarette.

Neuroscientists now think that the insula is the wellspring of emotions like lust and disgust, pride and humiliation, guilt and atonement. It helps give rise to moral intuition, empathy and the capacity to respond emotionally to music.

Thus, if it is affected one can see how it could cause various personality and behavioural changes.

Sex difficulties

This really does cause most people concern. There can be anxiety about the ability to have sex, one's attractiveness to one's partner and fear of causing damage to the brain.

In general, most people who have made a good recovery after having a stroke will be able to resume sexual activity. Yet others may experience difficulties including:

- Problems with erections

- Problems in achieving orgasm

- Problems in ejaculating

- Lowered libido

- Less sensitivity

- Reduced vaginal lubrication

- Problems with fears if there are continence issues.

If any of these occur then the matter should be raised with your general practitioner, who can refer you on to a range of therapists and specialists, including a continence advisor, gynaecologist, urologist and neurologist. The good news is that there is often something that can be done.

It is quite common for the libido to be affected for a short period after a stroke, but usually it builds back to pre-stroke normality. This loss of libido is more common with right-sided hemisphere strokes.

Depression can affect the libido, but once it is diagnosed and treated the libido may well improve.

Regarding whether it is safe to resume a sex life, the answer is that for most people who have had an ischaemic stroke it is probably OK to resume activity as soon as you feel comfortable. Patients who have had a haemorrhage, however, should consult with their general practitioner first.

People are often too embarrassed to talk about their love life, yet there is no reason why one should be troubled talking to one's partner.

Someone who has had a stroke has not become a different person; they will still be attractive to their partner. It may be that there will have to be some give and take and perhaps alteration in sexual positions, but a sex life can be resumed as long as it is acceptable to both. If the partner who had the stroke has been left with one side paralysed or reduced in sensation then it may be helpful to concentrate attention on the sensitive, unaffected side.

And if it is decided that active sex is not what they want then there is nothing wrong with simply enjoying a loving relationship with lots of hugs and kisses.

The important point is not to be embarrassed about asking for help.

Epilepsy

Some patients may develop epilepsy for a while after a stroke. This might become permanent if there is a persisting area of scar or infarction in the brain that acts to trigger off a wave of electricity throughout the brain.

A wave of electrical activity is the cause of a convulsion or a seizure – this can vary immensely, but often manifests as an episode of brief loss of attention, as if the individual is simply lost in thought. The individual is usually unaware that they have had such an episode but in some it is followed by slight confusion or even memory loss.

Others may have a full-blown convulsion in which they lose consciousness, fall to the ground with their limbs trembling. If such a convulsion is observed then the patient should be monitored, and any furniture near them should be moved back. False teeth should be removed to prevent choking, but do not make heroic attempts to stop the patient from swallowing their tongue. This is not necessary and will possibly do more harm than good.

Once the convulsion is over, put them into the recovery position, taking great care if they are paralysed on one side, and make them comfortable until they recover. If they seem to have had a second stroke, then you should summon help.

KEY POINTS

- Five per cent of stroke survivors will have an epileptic attack after a stroke.
- Few will require regular anti-epileptic medication in the long term.

Visual problems

Vision involves the function of the eyes and the brain. Visual problems are not uncommon with strokes, but they can be exceedingly complex to diagnose and to treat, since it depends upon which parts of the brain are affected. For example, if the cranial nerves are affected then the movements of the eyes can be impaired, resulting in blurring and double vision; and if the pathways inside the brain are affected, then the visual fields may be disturbed. If the parts of the brain that perceive vision are damaged, then this can produce visual neglect, or the phenomenon in which the person loses awareness of one half of the body or of anything that happens on that side. They can also lose depth sense and have immense problems in reaching for objects.

It is important to do as much as one can to help anyone who develops a visual problem as a result of their stroke.

KEY POINT

- Visual problems are most common in people who have strokes affecting the right side of the brain.

Vision

The eye is basically a spherical camera. The muscular sclera (the white of the eye) forms the sphere and is continuous with the transparent front of the eye, the cornea. Light rays enter the eye and are focused by the lens onto the retina, which is the light-sensitive 'seeing' membrane at the back of the eye. The amount of light let into the eye is determined by the reflex actions that govern the movement of the iris, and the shape of the lens and the focus are adjusted by the ciliary muscles. There are two fluids in the eye, the aqueous humour at the front of the eye and the jelly-like vitreous humour behind the lens.

The retina has two types of cells, called rods and cones. There are about 120 million rods in the eye and about 6 to 7 million cones, which are colour-sensitive. The rods are distributed about the whole retina, but the cones are predominantly situated around the centre of the retina, the part called the macula.

We track things with our eyes by moving the eyeball. Each eyeball has six muscles which work in harmony to allow us to move the eye in any direction. There are three cranial nerves on each side of the brain which operate these muscles.*

Signals from the eye are transmitted back to the brain via the optic nerve, which is the second of the 12 cranial nerves. The nerve

---

* Cranial nerve III, the oculomotor nerve which supplies four muscles; Cranial nerve IV, the trochlear nerve and Cranial nerve VI, the Abducens nerve, each of which supplies one muscle

consists of nerve fibres which actually carry the signals. One half of these fibres comes from the inner or nasal side of the retina and one half comes from the outer or temporal side of the retina. The two optic nerves join at a point called the optic chiasma. There, the fibres from the outer half of each eye pass directly along the optic pathway that leads to the visual cortex at the back of the brain via optic radiations (see Figure 7). The fibres from the inner halves of the retina cross over to the opposite side and travel along with the fibres from the outer half of the opposite eye.

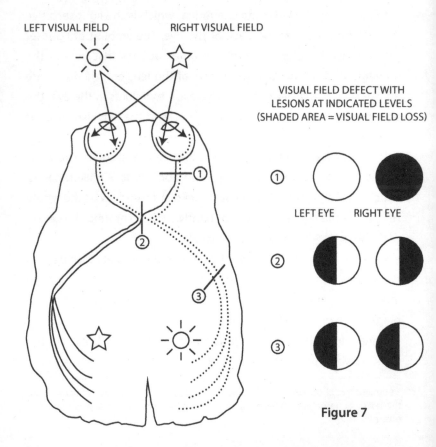

Figure 7

The visual field is the name that we give to the whole of what we see. Yet, like the image formed in a camera, it is actually an upside down and reversed image. The visual cortex then does an amazing thing. It turns the image formed by the camera of the eye the right way up and orientates it so that you see the world as it is.

Visual field loss

A stroke affecting one of the optic pathways may affect part of the vision in one or both eyes, as shown in Figure 7. This is called a hemianopia.

If half of both visual fields are affected by a stroke then it is called an homonymous hemianopia. If the right side of the visual field is affected it is called a right homonymous hemianopia and if the left side of the visual field is affected it is called a left homonymous hemianopia. This can cause a lot of difficulty, because the person cannot see either to the right or to the left, depending on which homonymous hemianopia they have. In reading, for example, a person with a right homonymous hemianopia will not see the end of sentences or words and a person with a left homonymous hemianopia will not see the beginnings. It can be incredibly frustrating.

This can be helped by the use of a typoscope, which is simply a card with a piece cut out which can be used to surround a word. An orthopist may also be able to teach the person a scanning technique. And various optical aids, including spectacles with prisms or small mirrors, may also be used.

Eye muscle problems

Eye muscle problems can arise if the third, fourth or sixth cranial nerves on either side are affected. This can lead to blurring of vision or double vision. An orthopist may be able to help by teaching exercises or using occlusion or patching over one eye, or by providing various types of prisms.

Nystagmus is a movement disorder that can be troublesome because the eye is subject to erratic little side-to-side movements which make focusing difficult. Once again, an orthopist may be able to advise.

Perception

A right-hemisphere stroke can cause more difficulties with vision, because it may affect the way that the brain processes perceptual information. A person may also have visual neglect, as mentioned earlier.

It may be possible to help the condition through exercises, visual aids and scanning techniques.

Dry eyes

This can be troublesome for some people if the blinking mechanism is affected or if the eyelid has been impaired so that the eye does not close properly. The eyeball will not be lubricated and can become very uncomfortable. Artificial tears prescribed by the doctor can help. The individual may need to be encouraged to try to blink more often.

Some people also experience increased sensitivity to light after a stroke and they may benefit from wearing tinted spectacles.

Amaurosis fugax

This is an episode of transient blindness in one eye, which can occur during a TIA. It is the result of interruption of the circulation to one eye caused by a blood clot from the heart or from narrowing of the carotid arteries in the neck. Some people experience a misting or a cloudiness in one eye, others experience full loss of vision in that eye. It may only last a few seconds or a few minutes.

This is not a symptom to be ignored. Like all TIAs it may herald the onset of a major stroke, so it should be dealt with urgently by a doctor.

Infections

Because the individual may have lost the ability to move one half of their chest the normal breathing system might be impaired. This may hamper the ability to raise the ribcage to help them inhale. In addition, they may not be able to move one side of their diaphragm, the sheet of muscle that separates the chest from the abdomen and which helps in breathing by acting like a bellows to suck air in during inspiration and force it out during expiration.

Any impairment of the swallow reflex may result in food or drink particles going down the wrong way and being inhaled. If the cough reflex is also impaired, the aspirated food or drink cause inflammation and act as a focus for infection. This is called aspiration pneumonia.

Raised temperature, a cough and shortness of breath are all indicative of a chest infection, which will probably require antibiotics to be prescribed. Severe chest infections can be life threatening.

Urinary infections are also more common after a stroke, because the function of the bladder may be impaired. This can result in stagnation of urine and infection can develop. Urinary infections are more likely if the bladder is catheterised.

Pain and stinging on passing urine and an increased desire to pass urine are symptoms that necessitate a sample of urine being checked for evidence of infection. If present an appropriate antibiotic should be given.

Pain

A stroke itself does not usually cause pain. Sometimes, however, parts of the brain are affected, which leaves the individual feeling pain in the parts of the body that were affected by the stroke. This pain is not usually sharp or acute, but is often described as dull, aching or numbing, as if it is deep inside the affected part of the body. It can be constant or it can come and go; it can certainly be quite distressing and hard to deal with. In some patients, painkillers do not seem to help.

This sort of chronic pain seems to come about when the human pain matrix is affected. This is a relatively recently-discovered mechanism by which we perceive and process pain.

The pain matrix

The pain matrix is a concept in medicine about the way that we perceive pain. Rather than the old idea that pain was transmitted up the spinal cord from a part of the body, like a wire leading directly to a higher part of the brain, it is now thought that there is a matrix, or a whole network of ways that nerve impulses can be passed up. This matrix seems to have two main components in the brain, which operate in unison with each other.

The lateral pain system seems to be responsible for processing the physical sensations, such as intensity of pain and its localisation. It has much to do with acute pain, such as the pain you feel when part of the body is traumatised.

The medial pain system processes the emotional side of pain. It passes its information up medially (on the inside) and it does it through our old friend the limbic system. The information is then passed up to the prefrontal cortex.

If the limbic system is affected by stroke it can cause a significant emotional memory to be associated with the sensation of pain.

Chronic pain can affect a lot of people after stroke and we shall look at how it may be possible to develop strategies to cope with this in **Chapter 12, Using the Life Cycle to come to terms with a stroke**.

KEY POINT

- Up to 75 per cent of stroke survivors face some form of pain as a result.

Specific pain problems

Shoulder pain is extremely common and relates to how that side was affected by a stroke. The muscles will be in a weakened state as recovery progresses. There may also have been problems with posture and with secondary damage to the joint when the side was paralysed.

As mentioned in the last chapter the stroke unit care will aim to minimise this problem, and good physiotherapy advice and appropriate aids should help.

Venous thromboembolism

Venous thromboembolism (VTE) is the name given to the development of a blood clot forming in the lower limb or pelvic veins. Such a clot is called a deep vein thrombosis, commonly referred to as a DVT. The danger is if this clot fragments and produces an embolus (a clot that is carried along in the blood stream), it may be carried to the lungs, where it can lodge in a blood vessel – with potentially catastrophic results. This is called a pulmonary embolism (PE).

Virchow's triad

The German physician Rudolph Virchow (1821–1902) was the first person to deduce the link between a DVT and a PE. He also formulated a triad of conditions that make venous thrombus formation more likely:

1. Damage to the inner lining of the vein

2. Venous stasis or stagnation of the blood from immobility

3. Abnormality of the clotting mechanism.

Stroke survivors are at definite risk of having a DVT by virtue of having paralysed muscles and being immobile as a result. If they become dehydrated then this can increase the coagulability or clotting tendency in the blood.

This is again where the expertise of the stroke unit is vital to prevent this complication.

KEY POINTS

- 20 per cent of untreated DVTs will develop a PE.
- In the UK, 25,000 people die each year from VTE: a greater number than the combined figures of deaths due to breast cancer, accidents and AIDS.[9]

Dementia

Each stroke has the potential to cause damage to the brain. In some patients who have repeated small strokes this can lead to multiple infarcts. This can significantly affect the cognitive ability of the individual and result in multi-infarct dementia, which is the second most common type of dementia after Alzheimer's disease.

Death

Stroke is the third most common cause of death in the UK.

Chapter 9

Aids and equipment for independent living

After a stroke the things that one took for granted – the movements and tasks of daily life – may present marked difficulties. One may not be able to walk unaided or perform complex movements, balance without support or be able to use one side of the body. A right-handed person may lose the use of their right side and have to learn to deal with everything using the left hand. The problem is that so many things are not designed for a left-handed user.

Washing, dressing, cooking may all be activities that become extremely difficult.

Usually a health and social care assessment will have been performed before discharge from hospital. Social services may be involved in this, liaising with the occupational therapist who performs the visit, so that they can act on the occupational therapist's recommendations. This is sometimes also referred to as a community care assessment. If, by chance, it was not arranged then you can request one.

The purpose of this assessment is twofold. It is to assess the suitability of the home for the stroke survivor and the carer. They may recommend that aids, special equipment or some adaptations to the home may need to be made.

The GP will be the main professional to see the patient after discharge from hospital and will liaise with district nurses, social services, physiotherapists and continence advisors, depending upon what the needs of the individual seem to be.

Some aids and adaptations may be available from social services through various grants, other things may need to be purchased from other agencies. The Stroke Association is very good at advising on this and it also has a facility whereby certain aids and equipment may be purchased.

Standing, walking and mobility

Adequate footwear may be needed to help provide a person with better support. The physiotherapist or occupational therapist may advise about:

- Hand-rails

- Fitting a stair-lift

- The need for a wheelchair

- Using walking sticks or a Zimmer frame.

Wheelchairs

A wheelchair may be necessary for some stroke survivors. There are different types of wheelchair – the most common ones are attendant (push) wheelchairs and self-propelled wheelchairs.

Powered wheelchairs, of which there are four types, are also available.

If a wheelchair is necessary, then you certainly need advice from your doctor or occupational therapist; they can refer you to the NHS Wheelchair Service, that can make an assessment of your needs and discuss funding options, if you are deemed eligible. There are variations according to local referral methods, since some areas operate a self-referral system.

You can check local situations on www.wheelchairmanagers.nhs.uk

The British Red Cross Medical Equipment service is a volunteer-led service that provides wheelchair short-term loans from almost 1,000 outlets in the UK. This can be extremely useful in those early days after discharge from hospital, but note that this is for short-term loans only.

www.redcross.org.uk

Daily living equipment

Many people who have had a stroke dislike the idea of having to use an aid or some sort of special equipment. There is no reason to feel this way, since these aids and pieces of equipment are simply tools. We all use tools in daily work and life, whether they are hammers, forceps, knitting needles or laptops.

Daily living equipment includes all sorts of aids, or tools, which can be used to help you do tasks that have started to become difficult as a result of a medical condition.

There are four types of daily living equipment:

1. Items for people with a significant disability to help them overcome a particular difficulty, e.g. a wheelchair, mobility aids, a bath board or a raised toilet seat, a step-in shower.

2. Standard equipment, or labour-saving devices, that can be used to ease the effort of a particular task, such as a food processor which removes the need to chop vegetables, an electric tin-opener instead of a manual one, a vacuum cleaner.

3. Standard equipment that has been modified, such as long-handled hairbrush or comb, long-handled spoons, special grips for cutlery for those who have difficulty with holding utensils.

4. Custom-made equipment for the individual to overcome a problem that is unique to them. This may include special left-sided gadgets or aids.
   See Anything Left-handed at www.anythingleft-handed.co.uk.

The Stroke Association operates Strokeshop which sells a range of products that may be of great help.
   Stroke Association House, 240 City Road, London, EC1V 2PR
   Phone: 020 7566 0300; Fax: 020 7490 2686; Textphone: 020 7251 9096. Their stroke helpline is open Monday to Friday, 9 a.m. to 5 p.m.: 0303 303 3100
   www.stroke.org.uk/contact

Personal alarms

Many people who have had a stroke feel vulnerable and may be at risk from falls. A personal alarm, linked to a community alarm scheme, is an alarm linked to a pendant that one wears or attached to a telephone. If the person finds they are in trouble they can activate the alarm which goes through to a local authority or district authority centre, where help can be mobilised.

There are differences about how these are organised in England and Wales, Northern Ireland and Scotland. Some housing authorities also run such schemes.

Chapter 10

Life after a stroke

Adapting the home

If it is decided and agreed that the stroke survivor is able to return home then it may be that some further adaptations, aside from daily living aids, will need to be made to the home. The Health and Social Care Assessment by the occupational therapist or physiotherapist will probably have highlighted the sort of things that could be done to help the person manage. This may relate to both inside and outside the home. It may be that circumstances change, perhaps because of a further problem developing, or because not all changes have been made. Or simply, the changes that were initially made are not adequate and do not significantly help.

All changes do need careful consideration and the stroke survivor needs to be involved in the decision-making wherever possible. In particular, it may be sensible to change the bedroom from upstairs to downstairs, rather than embarking on an expensive stair lift.

The carer may also, at a later stage, request an assessment, especially if they were not involved in the original assessment.

The following are common adaptations that may be needed:

- Widening of doorways and passageways, especially if a wheelchair or a walking aid like a Zimmer frame is going to be needed

- Moving light switches, doorbells, cupboard and door handles, and telephones

- Appropriate grab rails

- Arranging a downstairs toilet

- Adapting toilet and bathrooms – altering sink heights, back rests for the toilet, walk-in showers, power lifts to get in and out of the bath

- Powered hoists

- Levelling drives and paths

- Arranging internal and external ramps

- Stair lifts

- Special furniture – e.g. reclining chairs and electric controls to alter height.

Disabled facilities grant

Local authorities may be able to help with a Disabled Facilities Grant to make a home more suitable for someone with a permanent disability. Grants require the recommendation of an occupational therapist and are means-tested (entitlement to them is affected by the amount of income and savings that the individual has). They can be awarded to both owners and tenants of private or social dwellings, up to a maximum of £25,000.

The stroke survivor or their carer should contact the local authority.

Other important issues

There are several important areas that often cause stroke survivors a great deal of anxiety. Some of these areas, such as ability to drive or information about sex life, may have been touched upon when the person was in hospital but, if they were not covered, be sure to ask for advice. The general practitioner may be the first port of call.

Driving

Driving is another area of concern for many people after a stroke. You may need to inform the DVLA (the Driver and Vehicle Licensing Agency) in England, Wales and Scotland, or the DVA (the Driver Vehicle Agency) in Northern Ireland.

The DVLA produces a fact sheet which outlines its rules and recommendations for car or motorcycle drivers who have had a stroke or TIA.

KEY POINTS

- It is the stroke survivor's responsibility to inform the DVLA about any condition affecting driving ability.
- There is a fine of up to £1,000 if the DVLA is not informed.
- If you don't inform the DVLA and you have an accident you could be prosecuted.

The situation may change, but these are the current recommendations:

Anyone holding a bus, coach or lorry licence who has had a stroke must inform the DVLA, and they need to fill in form STR1V. You cannot drive and you will not be able to drive such a vehicle for a year. A medical report will be necessary first.

Anyone holding a car or motorcycle licence should not drive for one month. You then only have to inform the DVLA if you have persisting problems affecting the ability to drive. You need your general practitioner to agree that you are fit to drive.

The things that affect your fitness to drive are:

- Physical symptoms affecting the arms or legs, including weakness, paralysis, muscle spasms and sensory changes

- Visual problems, including blurred vision, loss of central vision in one or both eyes and visual field losses

- Cognitive effects, if your ability to think and concentrate is affected

- Fatigue

- Epilepsy, if it starts after a stroke. You cannot drive and you will have to be free of fits for a year

- Post carotid endarterectomy (see **Chapter 5, When a stroke strikes**). You will be able to drive after about three weeks, provided that you can perform an emergency stop. It is as well to double check with the DVLA and your general practitioner.

Insurance

Again, it is your responsibility to inform your insurance company, otherwise it may well not cover you in the event of an accident.

Blue badge

You may be entitled to a blue badge, which is a scheme that operates throughout the country. If you have restricted mobility it may be possible to get a badge which entitles you to park close to a destination using specially designated areas of streets or car parks. You have to apply to the local authority and your general practitioner may be able to support your application.

Mobility centres

These can assess your driving and advise about vehicle adaptations that may help you to drive. See Motability in Benefits, below.

Benefits

If you are still of working age, but unable to work at all, then you may be eligible for Personal Independence Payment (PIP). This benefit is to help towards some of the extra costs arising from a health condition or disability. It is based on how a person's condition affects them, not the condition they have.

Claimants can receive PIP whether they are in or out of work. The benefit is not means tested or taxed.

There are two components to PIP – for daily living and mobility needs. Each component can be paid at standard rate, or enhanced rate for those with the greatest needs.

PIP will include an assessment of the individual's needs by a health professional. Most people will have a face-to-face consultation as part of their claim.

For more information you can call Benefit Enquiry line 0800 882 200 Monday to Friday, 8 a.m. to 6 p.m.

Other benefits

If your income is much reduced following illness, you could look at a number of 'low income benefits'. Entitlement is based on the joint income of you and your partner if you are a couple, and will take account of any savings you may have:

- Income Support – extra help if your income is very low

- Housing Benefit – help towards rent which can be claimed from your local council

- Council Tax Benefit – help towards rent from your local council

- Tax credits – usually available if you or your partner are still working, but on a low income.

From October 2013, many of these low income benefits will be replaced with a new benefit called Universal Credit. It will replace: income-based Jobseeker's Allowance, income-related Employment and Support Allowance, Income Support, Child Tax Credits, Working Tax Credits and Housing Benefit.

Motability

The Motability Scheme enables disabled people to exchange either their Higher Rate Mobility Component of Disability Living Allowance or their War Pensioners' Mobility Supplement to obtain a new car, powered wheelchair or scooter.

Carer's Allowance

Currently, this is a weekly benefit to help a carer look after someone with substantial caring needs. The carer does not have to be related or living with the person. To obtain it you need to be aged over 16 years and spend at least 35 hours a week caring for them.

You need to be aware that it could affect other benefits, so check with the Benefit Enquiry line: 0800 882 200.

Carer's Credit

If you are looking after someone for at least 20 hours a week you could get Carer's Credit, which helps you build up entitlement to the basic State Pension and additional State Pension. Essentially it makes sure that there are no gaps in your National Insurance record.

Your income, savings or investments will not affect eligibility for Carer's Credit.

Disabled Person's Railcard

If you are unable to drive, but are able to use trains, then you may be able to obtain a Disabled Person's Railcard, which entitles you to a third off the fare.

Free bus pass

If you have a disability after a stroke, such as difficulty walking, or are partially sighted or blind, you may be able to obtain a free bus pass. This depends upon the rules in your locality.

A cautionary note

The benefit system is liable to change from time to time and so it is sensible to check with the Benefit Enquiry Helpline to get up-to-date information on benefits that are available:

Freephone: 0800 882 200

Textphone: 0800 243 355

Monday to Friday, 8 a.m. to 6 p.m.

www.gov.uk/benefit-enquiry-line/

Chapter 11

On becoming a carer

When a stroke occurs it does not simply affect the individual who has it, but will probably affect the whole family and whoever finds themselves in the role of carer. It may not be a long-term commitment if the stroke is recoverable to the extent that the person can live totally independently. However, since one-third of all strokes leave people with permanent disability of some degree, it means that many people will become dependent upon a carer or a family.

Currently, there are about six million carers in the UK – to put this in context, about one in every six households has a carer.

Carer's assessment

We mentioned this in the section about the home assessment. In fact, the person who becomes the carer for a stroke survivor may not have been involved while the stroke person was in hospital. If this is the case, then a carer's assessment can be requested if the person that needs caring is eligible for social services help.

The aim of this is to assess what support the carer needs in order to maintain their own health and wellbeing.

Carers Direct

This is an official website that is a treasure trove of information that can help the carer get help and support: www.nhs.uk/CarersDirect/carerslives/updates/Pages/new-to-carers-direct.aspx

You can also call the Carers Direct helpline on 0808 802 0202.

This is open Monday to Friday from 9 a.m. to 8 p.m. and from 11 a.m. to 4 p.m. on Saturday and Sunday.

There you can find information about:

- Your rights

- Benefits

- Direct payments

- Leaving work or returning to work or education

- Advice on getting a carer's assessment

- Housing issues

- Home care.

Getting into a routine

When one begins caring it can seem very confusing. It is important, therefore, to try to establish a routine; this can be based upon the stroke survivor's needs. A useful thing to do is to keep a diary over a week so that you can chart the tasks that you need to get done, when and where and how much time they take.

The aim of this is not to load yourself down with tasks, but to see what you can do to help the person you are caring for become more independent. It may help you to define what aids and services can be asked for in order to help.

Continuing to work with the community team

Once the patient is at home the stroke team will probably keep in touch for a while, then hand on care to the community team. It is important that, if the stroke survivor needs such help, the carer has been shown how to lift effectively and safely. They will be shown how to do this by the physiotherapist and occupational therapist.

The GP will be the person that you liaise with in the community team and who will look after the stroke survivor's medical care and mobilise whatever other help is needed. This may include help from:

- Nurse practitioner or practice nurse

- District or community nurse

- Continence advisor

- Physiotherapist

- Speech therapist

- Health visitor

- Pharmacist

- Social worker.

Looking after yourself

Very often a carer, whether a husband, wife, sibling or child, will end up taking on many other tasks, such as cooking, bathing, lifting, organising finances and overseeing the administration of medication. It can be physically demanding and emotionally draining. It is important, therefore, to allow yourself free time, adequate time to eat and to sleep.

Stress can be a problem so it is useful to seek advice from your general practitioner if you develop a sleep problem, experience anxiety attacks or develop any physical symptoms.

It is also as well to be aware of what coping mechanisms you use to ease stress and see how your use of them can be improved or optimised. Some carers lean on habits or coping mechanisms that may be injurious to their health – smoking and drinking are obvious ones, but so too are things like gambling, eating junk food or becoming less active. In other words, some coping mechanisms are better than others. In the next chapter we shall look at a simple means of drawing things together that I call the Life Cycle. It is not rocket science, but it gives a means of developing various strategies that may help.

Day care and respite care

Since caring can be physically, emotionally and psychologically draining, day care may have been organised as part of a package of care. This is usually in a residential or nursing home, depending upon how much care the stroke survivor needs.

Respite care is effectively a longer period of care for a week or two for the stroke patient in a residential or nursing home or a local hospital. If it is available then you as the carer should take the opportunity to rest or do whatever you need to recharge the batteries.

Stroke clubs and carers' groups

If they are available locally, stroke clubs are very helpful for stroke survivors to attend. They give the carer regular time off from their care work, so that they can get on with other tasks and get some respite. They are also of great benefit to the stroke survivor, since they give a social outlet where rehabilitation can continue.

Carers' groups may also be available where a carer can meet other carers, share experiences and receive support. This can be of inestimable value, since many people find themselves suddenly put into a caring role after a relative, spouse or partner has a stroke. The new carer may feel ill-equipped to take the role on; they may feel angry at having it thrust upon them, or they may find themselves becoming ill as a result of the stress. Talking to other people who are in the same position or who have experienced similar problems can help by allowing the new carer to learn from others' experience. It always helps to know that you are not alone.

Very often one can establish new friends, new contacts who can be built up into a support network of people that you can contact to talk through a problem.

Change of relationship

Being a carer to a relative or partner can alter the relationship markedly. It may mean taking over responsibilities that were always the other person's, or having to perform duties that you find intrusive or which alter the way in which you perceive one another. These things take time to get accustomed to and it is not unusual to find oneself experiencing changing emotions. Some people become closer, others develop irritability and resentment, others feel guilty.

Your GP is always someone that you should be able to discuss these issues with, but here again you may find a local carers' group of great benefit. Other people will have been through the same things and their experiences may help you to deal with how you are feeling.

Of course, it may be that the way that you are feeling might need treatment if you are feeling anxious or depressed. Your doctor in that case may decide to prescribe or arrange some counselling.

Never refuse help

This is important. People will often offer help soon after a stroke, but if it is turned down, because the carer thinks that they can cope or because they feel in some way embarrassed about accepting help, then further offers may not be made. Another reason that people refuse help is because they do not want to feel obligated to anyone else. There is no need to feel this, since the offer was clearly a friendly and concerned gesture. Accept it in this light and you will maintain a contact that may be very useful later on.

There is nothing to be embarrassed or guilty about. Maintain all the contacts that you can, accept help if it is offered, even if it is simply a matter of someone collecting a newspaper, doing a few errands, or changing a light bulb.

Chapter 12

Coming to terms with a stroke – using the Life Cycle

Having a stroke can have a huge impact both upon the individual and their family. It is often easy to get locked into a way of thinking and focus all of one's attention on one or two aspects of the condition. Yet by looking at all areas of one's life and how they are impacted upon you may be able to develop strategies that help.

One way of doing this is by considering the different spheres of one's life. The following simple model may help to 'see' how one can develop strategies to help.

The Life Cycle

This heading may take you back to your days of studying biology when you looked at the different life cycles of insects, fish, frogs and other creatures on the evolutionary ladder. In fact, used in the sense that I am going to outline, it does not have anything to do with the individual's development or with their medical history leading up to having a stroke. It is simply a way of looking at one's life in the here and now.

The Life Cycle is to do with the different levels or spheres that make up one's life now. And you will see that there is a cycle involved, certainly in the manner in which a condition, virtually any chronic medical condition, can affect them.

Yet to use the biology analogy a little longer, you will learn a certain amount about fish by dissecting them to look at their internal organs, but you won't know how they move and feed without studying them in water. And you won't learn about their behaviour with other fish and predators unless you observe them in a realistic environment. Even then, you will not get to know about them fully unless you just become a total observer of them.

So it is in medicine. In order to help someone you need to know as much as possible about their condition, their symptoms and the things that make their symptoms better or worse. And, ideally, you want to know about their habits, their diet, their desires, their fears, their relationships and so on. That might seem like a tall order, but if you can build up such a picture of the person, then you can see how a condition is truly affecting them throughout all levels of their life.

There are five levels or spheres of life that we need to consider:

Body – what symptoms you have, e.g. pain, stiffness, weakness of a limb, tiredness.

Emotions – how does it make you feel, e.g. anxious, sad, depressed, angry or jealous of others who are not affected.

Mind – how it affects the type of thoughts you have, e.g. pessimistic thoughts, negative thoughts, self-defeating thoughts.

Behaviour – how it makes you behave, e.g. isolating yourself by avoiding things or people. Or by developing habits, e.g. smoking, drinking, becoming inactive.

Lifestyle – how it affects your ability to do things, your relationships, and also how events in your life impact on you. It also relates to the effect that the stroke has upon your carer or carers and your family.

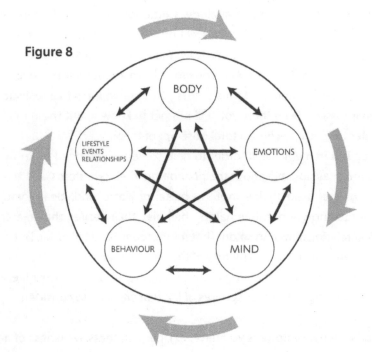

Figure 8

If you look at Figure 8 you will see that there is a circle for each of the five spheres and that these are interconnected by a series of outer arrows and inner arrows. Indeed, each sphere is connected to every other one by one or other arrow. This represents the way that any symptom can in fact have an effect on every aspect of your life. But equally, every other area or sphere of your life can have an impact on the one symptom. This may be very important, since it gives us the potential to build strategies to help deal with a stroke.

Chronic pain

As mentioned earlier in the book some people are left with a chronic or continuous pain problem after a stroke. To deal with the pain the person may have been prescribed painkillers and may take them regularly to keep the pain under control. Very often the painkiller is not enough and the dose may end up being increased, or different painkillers are used; the painkillers may constipate the person and then a laxative may be used. So it can become quite complex, in that other problems compound it. This tends to have a reinforcing effect on the pain.

Yet drugs are not the only means of dealing with pain. If you use the Life Cycle to view each of the five spheres you will get the idea.

Firstly, 'body' is about the physical symptom of pain. What sort of pain is it? Is it an aching pain, shooting pain, throbbing pain? Is it there all the time or does it come and go? What makes it better (e.g. heat or cold) and what makes it worse (e.g. movement, temperature change)?

Secondly, 'emotions' is about how this makes you feel. One can see that a chronic pain could affect the emotions and make one feel sad or depressed, angry or frustrated.

Thirdly, 'mind' refers to the sort of thoughts that go through one's mind. Are they negative thoughts like, 'Here we go again', or 'Why me?'

Fourthly, 'behaviour' means what does it make you do or what do you do about it? Do you rub the part? Do you reach for a painkiller or light up a cigarette or reach for a drink?

Fifthly, 'lifestyle' is linked to the behaviour and the habits you adopt, but it is also to do with what it does to your life, your relationship with your carer, your family and your friends. Does it make you withdraw, become isolated?

If it does make you isolated, how does that come about? Is it because you withdraw, or because you push people away, or because your actions make people withdraw from you? And in what ways does this happen?

These are not meant to be value judgements, just ways that you need to see how a symptom is affecting you.

So far we have followed the Life Cycle's outer sequence of arrows, seeing how the body symptoms affect the emotions, then how the emotions affect the thoughts and so on. But take any one sphere and look at the other arrows, which indicate that every other sphere is potentially affected by that pain. That means that the pain may well have affected the individual in that outer sequential manner, but also it gives you, via the inner arrows, various possible strategies that may modify the pain.

In **Chapter 8, Complications after a stroke**, we mentioned the pain matrix, the neurological network that is involved in the perception of pain. Chronic pain seems to get routed via the limbic system, which is associated with emotions. Thus, chronic pain will have an emotional content and, as a result of the emotional memory being triggered, it may well be associated with a particular chain of thoughts that come to mind. Thus, the pain triggers the emotion of anxiety – 'Oh dear, here is that awful pain again. The only thing to do is to take a painkiller'.

In other words, a negative emotion and a negative thought and the resultant behaviour is triggered. This is not to say that the action of taking a painkiller is a negative behaviour. It *may* be the right thing to do, but it is not always the right thing to do.

If, instead of allowing the negative emotion and the negative thought to come to the fore, the individual can think a positive thought, such as 'The pain will go away soon', whilst at the same time trying think of a happy image or event, and doing something totally different like pruning the roses, starting a crossword or making a cup of tea, then the action of taking a painkiller may not be needed or acted upon.

Success begets success and if this distraction works once it will work again.

And this method can be used to focus on the whole situation or upon any symptom or behaviour that you would like to modify.

Develop positive thinking

If you are of a pessimistic nature then you are more likely to get depressed, feel anxious, experience more pain and even have a higher risk of conditions like heart disease and cerebrovascular disease. You are also more likely to pick up colds and other respiratory infections.

It is thought that this is in part due to a psycho-neuro-immunological (PNI) mechanism. This refers to the growing realisation that the mind (psyche), the nervous system (neuro) and the immune (immuno) system are all interconnected. Thus stress can affect the nervous system and thence the immune system. A lot of stress can throw a strain on the whole system, so that the immune system works below par and one can pick up an infection.

We all operate these PNI mechanisms to varying degrees and you can have positive PNI mechanisms and negative ones. A positive one is seen in people who are able to delay an illness, but who then go down with something on the first day of their holiday. A negative one is seen when some stress is immediately followed by an illness. This can take one out of the work environment.

Pessimists are more likely to operate the negative PNI mechanisms and optimists the positive ones.

Logotherapy

Let me tell you about this quite remarkable therapy, which was developed by a remarkable man. I first came across it when I was working in psychiatry at the start of my medical career.

Viktor Frankl was the founder of a system of psychiatry known as 'logotherapy'. This is sometimes referred to as the 'Third Viennese School of Psychiatry'. Sigmund Freud's psychoanalysis is accepted as being the first, and Alfred Adler's Individual psychology was the second. Frankl had developed his theories during stays in three concentration camps, including the dreaded Auschwitz.

In establishing his philosophy of logotherapy, Frankl established three basic beliefs: firstly, that life has meaning under all circumstances, even the most miserable ones; secondly, that our main motivation is our will to find meaning in life; thirdly, that we have freedom to find meaning in what we do and what we experience.

The essence of all this is that we have choice as to how we view things. One must work against a tendency to be pessimistic and to try to become an optimist. To begin with, you have to consider self-talk. This is the name that we give to the endless stream of thoughts that runs through your head every day. Pessimists, who may be more prone to depression, tend to have a lot of negative automatic thought. Let me give you four examples of such negative thought:

Filtering – is where the individual filters out all the positives and sees only the negative. For example, despite a good day at work, they focus on the single error.

Personalisation – whenever something goes wrong they automatically assume it is their fault.

Catastrophising – they extrapolate all situations to the worst scenario, usually finding a reason for not doing something in order to prevent a supposed humiliation risk.

Polarisation – they see everything as two poles, good or bad, black or white, with nothing between.

To think positively, you have to monitor your self-talk and try to alter the negativity. For example, instead of thinking 'I can't do it because I have never done it before', try thinking, 'It's an opportunity to learn'. Or instead of 'There is no way this will work for me', try 'Let me try to make this work'.

This is all very relevant to the Life Cycle, because if you allow yourself to become pessimistic then you will get into a particular mind-set. You will affect your emotions and tend to get anxious and depressed. And this in turn will mean that you tend to adopt particular behaviour patterns.

Returning to the example of pain, if you anticipate that you are going to have a pain, you may end up taking more painkillers. And you may end up taking them when you do not actually need them. An optimist, on the other hand, may feel that it will go away if they do something else, that is, adopt another behaviour pattern and distract themselves, which as we have seen can make matters easier.

Anticipatory anxiety and paradoxical intention

One of the most important of Frankl's concepts was that of anticipatory anxiety. This is actually more than simply the fear that one has before an event. It is the anxiety about something happening, which is actually likely to make it happen. In logotherapy a technique of 'paradoxical intention' is used instead.

Take insomnia, for example. If you are an insomniac you usually go to bed and try too hard to sleep, the result being that you cannot sleep. With paradoxical intention you try to do the exact opposite. That is, you go to bed and you try 'not to sleep'. You may be amazed at how hard it then is to stay awake.

Another example is during an attack of hiccups. Instead of trying to stop them, try to make yourself hiccup. Offer yourself £10 to hiccup again. This paradoxical intention method usually makes them just stop.

The reason is that the fear in anticipation, the 'anticipatory fear', builds and builds until it becomes a far greater issue than the thing one is fearful of. Often, doing the opposite of what you feel you should do will remove the fear and when it has gone, so does the problem about the thing you were worried about. This happens because doing the opposite will seem to be a move that produces a situation that could be much worse than the original. With the problem of not sleeping, for example, by trying to stay awake you would be trying to do the very thing that you don't want to happen. It is greater in the mind than the fear of not sleeping.

So, the aim with paradoxical intention is to do something that you would think would worsen the problem – but it doesn't.

Let us look at a couple of case histories to see how this can be applied.

A 52-year-old man woke in the night with a sudden, excruciating headache. His wife awoke to the sound of him retching out of the bed. He told her that his head felt as if it was bursting and he slumped unconscious over the side of the bed.

She called 999 and managed to roll him onto his side and made sure that he did not choke. By the time the paramedics arrived he had regained consciousness, but could not move, because any movement increased the pain in his neck and head. He was admitted to accident and emergency and then to a neurosurgery ward where a diagnosis of a subarachnoid haemorrhage was made. He had weakness down his left side, although not paralysis.

He recovered well over several weeks but started to have convulsions within the first two days in hospital. He was also told that he had bled from a small aneurysm, but that he had another one in a place that was inaccessible to surgery. No treatment for it was possible and the rest of his management would concern the treatment of his epilepsy, for which he was referred to neurologists.

He left hospital after three weeks on several anticonvulsants. The epilepsy was difficult to control and the medication had to be increased. He was unable to drive, lost his job and became profoundly depressed. The choice of anti-depressant caused some problem, since it was believed that they could worsen his epilepsy. When one was finally chosen he experienced only partial improvement in his depression.

He became quite withdrawn and admitted that he felt as if he was living under the sword of Damocles, in constant fear. The knowledge that he had a large inoperable aneurysm that could burst at any time made him feel that he was living on borrowed time.

The pressure was thrown on his wife, who felt frustrated that he was unwilling to do more for himself. She felt that he had given up.

The Life Cycle applied

Together with his wife, the man was encouraged to make an entry on paper for each of the spheres of the Life Cycle. By simply drawing the five circles and linking them up with the arrows, and putting the list of symptoms inside the appropriate spheres they saw how each sphere could interact with the other. This then gave them the opportunity to see how they could try to modify each effect as it arose. Effectively, rather than, for example, taking a painkiller for a pain, they could look at ways that a body sensation such as pain could be modified by doing something to affect the emotions sphere, or the mind sphere or even the behaviour sphere.

Here is a listing of the spheres when they first thought about them:

Body
Fits
Headaches
Lack of erections

Emotions
Depressed
Black moods
Guilt

Mind
Think about bleak future
Never work again
Worry about my wife

Behaviour
Smoke
Throw things
Drink alcohol – even though advised not to

Lifestyle
It has gone!
Can't do anything
Lost sex drive
Lost self-esteem
Lost feeling that I am a man

Just looking at these problems, they can seem insurmountable. All is gloomy and each thing is negative. In fact, when they are put into the Life Cycle, one can see that they do all link up and that they do all contribute to how the patient was feeling. Interestingly, when they did their own Life Cycles, they put different things in the spheres, because that then gave them an idea of how the stroke was affecting both the individual and the carer.

You can see that the physical symptoms made him experience various negative emotions. This made him think and act in negative ways. It becomes a cycle of negativity and when you look at the internal arrows, each sphere impinged on the others.

That is all the explanation side of things. It is useful to help understand how the condition is affecting the individual and the family. The important point, however, is that the different spheres can all be used to offer different positive strategies that can be tried.

For example, instead of lighting up another cigarette when one thinks 'Oh blast it, I'm going to have a smoke', try to see how you can shift that negative feeling. The point is that the smoking is a behaviour that may have been triggered by the negative thought and by the negative emotion. What can you do in the emotional sphere, the mind sphere or the behaviour sphere to make you feel better?

Note also that in the body sphere he had put lack of erection and in the lifestyle lost sex drive. Some exploration on these issues showed that they were important to him, but because of them they contributed to lower his mood and made him use other negative behaviours, like the smoking and the alcohol. These of course did nothing but contributed further to the problem, as well as increased the risk to his further health.

Fear of bursting the aneurysm produced the sword of Damocles way of thinking and effectively shut off his libido and caused the erectile dysfunction. This is important, since some explanation that sex would be unlikely to burst his aneurysm helped him to see how he could devise other strategies to help. Specifically, reassurance from his neurologist on this count helped to dispel the fear.

Then, using paradoxical intention (see the section on logotherapy, and anticipatory anxiety and paradoxical intention), he was able, with the understanding of his wife, to rekindle his love life. The reassurance had helped, but by actually trying to make love he was able to restore his self-esteem as a man (his description) and remove his fear of rupturing the aneurysm.

This was done in a two-stage process. Firstly, he was able to restore his ability to have an erection by having a ban put on actually making love. Only foreplay was allowed until he could with confidence achieve an erection. This removed the anticipatory fear about failing to achieve an erection. Then, when the ban was lifted and successful sex life was regained, the other fears went and his self-esteem improved, allowing him to regain a sense of purpose in life.

A 70-year-old woman had a stroke while having dinner with her son and daughter-in-law. She was admitted to hospital and found to have a right hemisphere ischaemic stroke, from which she made a reasonable recovery, but which left her with a slight left-sided weakness. She had been a keen golfer, but her mobility was so reduced that she was unable to get back to her sport. She was also a keen crossword and Sudoku solver, but she found herself unable to concentrate on these any longer.

Her spheres were:

Body
Weakness
Limp
Difficulty with eating

Emotions
Frustration
Anger

Thoughts
I keep getting angry with myself
Tell my left hand to work for me

Behaviour
Become apathetic
Letting myself go

Lifestyle
Can't play golf
Can't do what I want
Withdrawing from my friends

With some thought she decided that the stroke was precluding her from playing golf but it would not stop her taking up new activities. She kept up her golf club membership as a social member and made herself go and play bridge once a week with friends at the club.

She also worked on her weakness with a mirror box and gradually improved the function of her left hand.

Yoga

One lifestyle change that seems to help people with strokes is yoga. One study published in the journal *Stroke* in 2012 followed up a group of men and women who had suffered from stroke. They divided the group into three groups as follows:

- A twice-a-week yoga group for eight weeks.
- A yoga-plus group that also had yoga twice a week, but with an additional relaxation session three times a week.
- A control group that had no yoga.

They found that the yoga groups showed significant improvements in their balance and were less afraid of falling. In addition, they had higher scores for independence and quality of life.

It is not all doom and gloom

There is no doubt that a stroke is a serious event, but most people do make a recovery sufficient to live independently. While they may need to adapt their lifestyle and do some mental readjustment, there is no reason that they cannot go on to lead a useful and enjoyable existence.

The Life Cycle approach is simply a means of seeing how different spheres of one's life impact on others. Because of that, you can work on any of them to produce an effect on any one that seems to be causing a problem.

Remember about brain plasticity, which we considered at the start of Part Two. The brain is always trying to reroute and find alternative pathways to transmit messages, so practising any exercises that have been given to you is always worthwhile.

Viktor Frankl's logotherapy and his ideas about anticipatory anxiety and paradoxical intention are worth keeping in mind. His three principles are worth restating:

1. Life has meaning under all circumstances, even the most miserable ones.

2. Our main motivation is our will to find meaning in life.

3. We have freedom to find meaning in what we do, and what we experience.

It is all too easy to become negative and to allow negative thoughts into one's mind, but strive to be an optimist. There are many things that you will be able to do and enjoy.

And finally, by aiming to incorporate lifestyle changes into your life to reduce the risk of having another stroke you will be taking positive steps to generally improve your health.

Your aim should be to keep well, stay positive and enjoy life to the best of your ability.

Glossary

ABCD² – an algorithm used to assess the risk of having a stroke after a TIA has been confirmed.

alteplase – a thrombolytic or clot-busting drug that may be given in an ischaemic stroke to break up a blood clot.

Alzheimer's disease – the most common form of dementia.

amaurosis fugax – temporary loss of vision in one eye as the result of a TIA.

anaphylactic reaction – a serious, potentially life-threatening allergic reaction characterised by low blood pressure, shock and difficulty breathing. It is a medical emergency.

angioplasty – a procedure in which a catheter is inserted into a groin artery and passed up into the neck arteries in order to inflate a small balloon to open up the vessel. It may be combined with placing a stent to keep the vessel open.

anticoagulant – a drug to prevent blood coagulation. Warfarin, rivaroxaban and dabigatran are examples.

antiplatelet – a drug, such as aspirin, which prevents platelets from sticking together.

apoplexy – archaic term for a stroke.

aspirin – the common name for acetylsalicylic acid, an antiplatelet agent that thins the blood and may be given to prevent a stroke.

arteriosclerosis – hardening of the arteries caused by accumulation of atheroma.

artery – blood vessel that carries oxygenated blood away from the heart, taking it to specific organs.

aspiration pneumonia – a dangerous situation when food or drink passes into the airway if the swallowing mechanism has been disrupted after a stroke.

atheroma – fatty changes in a blood vessel.

atrial fibrillation – an irregular beating of the heart caused by loss of the heart's normal pacemaker.

cardiovascular disease – disease affecting the heart and the blood vessels, which can result in heart attacks, strokes and death.

carotid endarterectomy – an operation performed to remove a thickened and narrowed stenosis in the carotid artery. However, there is a risk that the procedure could produce a stroke and less invasive treatments may be considered first.

cerebral embolism – when an embolus from the heart (usually from atrial fibrillation) lodges in a brain blood vessel to cause a stroke.

cerebral thrombosis – blood clot forming in a brain blood vessel.

cerebro-vascular accident CVA – old term for a stroke.

cerebro-vascular disease – disease of the blood supply to the brain.

CHADS$_2$ – an algorithmic check to assess risk of stroke in patients with non-valvular atrial fibrillation, and for considering the use of antiplatelet drugs like aspirin or anticoagulants.

Circle of Willis – the main blood supply to the brain.

clopidogrel – an antiplatelet agent that thins the blood and may be given to prevent a stroke.

COX enzymes – cyclo-oxygenase enzymes, involved in producing prostaglandins and thromboxane. Aspirin blocks their effect.

diabetes mellitus – a disorder of carbohydrate metabolism from too little insulin, or from a lack of response to the body's own insulin.

dipyridamole – an antiplatelet agent that thins the blood and may be given to prevent a stroke.

Doppler – a type of ultrasound scan.

DVT deep-vein thrombosis – the name for a thrombus or clot that forms in one of the deep veins of the lower limb.

embolism – the damage that occurs when an embolus lodges in a blood vessel. See cerebral embolism.

haemorrhagic stroke – a bleed into the brain.

hemianopia – loss of visual field.

homonymous hemianopia – loss of half of the visual field in each eye.

infarction – permanent damage to tissue after cells have died, to leave scar tissue.

INR (international normalised ratio) – a blood test used to check on the dosage of warfarin needed.

ischaemia – deprivation of tissue of oxygen.

ischaemic cascade – part of the pathological process that begins when brain cells are damaged in a stroke.

ischaemic stroke – a stroke that is caused by a disruption of the blood supply to the brain by a blockage from a thrombus or an embolism.

lacunar infarction – a specific type of death of brain cells, caused by blockage of a small, deep brain artery. It results in a melting away of brain tissue to produce a hole, like the hole in a sponge.

nasogastric tube – a tube passed up the nose into the stomach in order to deliver food and fluids.

necrosis – the process of cell and tissue death.

parenteral nutrition – feeding by intravenous means.

PEG tube – Percutaneous Endoscopically-placed Gastroenterostomy tube, used for feeding someone who is unable to swallow. It is placed into the stomach and emerges through the abdominal wall.

plaque – fatty streaks inside an artery. They may rupture, causing an inflammatory reaction and the start of a clot.

platelet – the smallest type of blood cell. It does not contain DNA. Its function is to clump with other platelets to form a clot to plug a bleeding vessel and help heal a wound.

prostaglandin – natural hormones that are involved in many body processes, including pain, tissue injury and inflammation.

pulmonary embolism – when an embolism from a DVT lodges in a lung vessel.

stenosis – a narrowing of an artery.

stent – a tiny wire tube that is placed inside a narrowed artery after an angioplasty in order to keep the vessel open.

stroke – brain attack as a result of a thrombosis, embolism or haemorrhage.

stroke in evolution – a gradually increasing cluster of symptoms over time as the stroke is continuing to evolve.

swallow test – a check that is done immediately upon admission or as soon as possible after a stroke to ensure that the swallowing mechanism is intact. If it is not, then food and drink must not be given.

thrombolytic drug – also known as a clot-buster, a drug that may be given in an ischaemic stroke to break down a clot.

thrombosis – the process of blood clotting.

thrombus – blood clot.

Transient Ischaemic Attack (TIA) – often called a mini-stroke. This is a brain attack, from which a complete recovery is made within 24 hours.

typoscope – a card with a piece cut out which can be used to surround a word.

vein – blood vessel that returns blood to the heart.

yoga – a system of exercises performed to promote control of body and mind.

Directory

Anything Left-handed

A group that provides products and information to make life easier for left-handed people. It has a mail-order business able to send products around the world.

www.anythinglefthanded.co.uk
Anything Left-Handed
PO Box 344
Tadworth KT20 9DL

Please note that they operate from a commercial warehouse and do not have a facility suitable for customer visits.

Telephone: 01737 888269

Benefit Enquiry Line

The Benefit Enquiry Line provides advice and information for disabled people and carers on the range of benefits available, including Attendance Allowance, Disability Living Allowance, Carer's Allowance, Carer's Credit and Universal Credit.

2nd Floor
Red Rose House
Lancaster Road
Preston
Lancashire PR1 1HB
Freephone: 0800 882 200

Textphone: 0800 243 355
Monday to Friday, 8 a.m. to 6 p.m.
www.gov.uk/benefit-enquiry-line/

British Red Cross
The British Red Cross Medical Equipment service is a volunteer-led service that provides wheelchair hire and short-term loan equipment at almost 1,000 outlets in the UK. This can be extremely useful in those early days after discharge from hospital.
You can find your local branch on:

www.redcross.org.uk

Citizens Advice Bureau (CAB)
The Citizens Advice Bureau aims to provide the advice people need for the problems they face and to improve the policies and practices that affect people's lives. The service provides free, independent and confidential advice. Advice by phone is available from all CAB and a national phone service is in development.

www.citizensadvice.co.uk
For England call 08444 111 444
For Wales call 08444 772 020
TextRelay users should call 08444 111 445

Disabled Living Foundation (DLF)
DLF is a national charity that provides impartial advice, information and training on daily living equipment.

380–384 Harrow Road
London W9 2HU
Helpline: 0845 130 9177

Textphone: 020 7432 8009
Email: helpline@dlf.org.uk

Drivers and Vehicle Licensing Agency (DVLA)

This organisation provides information about driving, licensing and medical conditions affecting driving. It is the organisation responsible for maintaining licences and provides information on all aspects of driving licences.

Drivers Medical Group
DVLA
Swansea SA99 1TU

Driver Licensing Enquiries

Telephone: 0300 790 6801
Textphone: 0300 123 1278
Fax: 0300 123 0784
Fax from outside the UK: +44 (0)1792 786 369
Monday to Friday, 8 a.m. to 7 p.m.; Saturday, 8 a.m. to 2 p.m.

Drivers Medical Enquiries

Telephone: 0300 790 6806 (car or motorcycle)
Telephone: 0300 790 6807 (bus, coach or lorry)
Fax: 0845 850 0095
Monday to Friday, 8 a.m. to 5.30 p.m.; Saturday, 8 a.m. to 1 p.m.

NHS Wheelchair Service

The Wheelchair Service provides appropriate mobility equipment for people of all ages with a long-term disability (i.e. likely to last longer than six months) who have difficulty in walking. They will help to choose a wheelchair that best meets the individual's needs.

There is usually provision for short-term loan wheelchairs (i.e. less than six months).

www.wheelchairmanagers.nhs.uk/services.asp

NICE
The National Institute for Health and Clinical Excellence was set up in 1999 to reduce variation in availability and quality of NHS treatment and care. NICE issues evidence-based guidance on the management of various conditions and public health guidance, recommending best ways to encourage healthy living, promote wellbeing and prevent disease. It is funded by the Department of Health.

www.nice.org.uk

The Chartered Society of Physiotherapy
The Chartered Society of Physiotherapy (CSP) is the professional, educational and trade union body for the UK's 49,000 chartered physiotherapists, physiotherapy students and assistants.

14 Bedford Row
London WC1R 4ED
Telephone: 020 7306 6666

The Royal National Institute of Blind People (RNIB)
RNIB is the leading charity offering information, support and advice to people with sight loss. It can offer practical ways to help live with sight loss and can advise to help people travel, shop and manage finances. They can also advise on technology for blind and partially sighted people.

It is a membership organisation that works with and for its membership.

RNIB Headquarters
105 Judd Street
London WC1H 9NE
Telephone: 0303 123 9999
Email: helpline@rnib.org.uk

Speakability

A UK charity dedicated to supporting and empowering people with aphasia and their carers. It offers impartial information and support through its helpline, website and training courses. It distributes its own factsheets, low-cost publications and DVDs.

Freephone: 080 8808 9572
Monday to Friday, 10 a.m. to 4 p.m. (answerphone at all other times)
Staff have been trained by the Telephone Helplines Association (THA)

Stroke Association

A UK charity dealing with stroke in people of all ages. It offers a one-off welfare grant for which a professional, e.g. GP, social worker or physiotherapist, must make an application. Its Stroke Information Service provides timely, accurate and personalised information.

Stroke House
240 City Road
London EC1V 2PR
Helpline: 0845 30 33 100 (local call rate) or 0303 30 33 100
Admin: 020 7566 0300
Fax: 020 7490 2686
www.stroke.org.uk

References

1 Lindhardsen J, Ahlehoff O, Gislason GH, et al. Risk of atrial fibrillation and stroke in rheumatoid arthritis: Danish nationwide cohort study. *BMJ* 2012; DOI:10.1136/bmj.e1257. Available at: www.bmj.com.

2 Fisher M, Lees K, Spence JD. Nutrition and stroke prevention. *Stroke* 2006; 37(9): 2430–2435.

3 Johnston SC, Rothwell PM, Nguyen-Huynh MN, Giles MF, Elkins JS, Bernstein AL, Sidney S. Validation and refinement of scores to predict very early stroke risk after transient ischaemic attack. *Lancet* 2007; 369: 283–292.

4 Stroke Unit Trialists' Collaboration. Organised inpatient (stroke unit) care for stroke. *Cochrane Database of Systematic Reviews* 2007 Oct 17; (4): CD000197.

5 Foley N, Salter K, Teasell R. Specialized stroke services: a meta-analysis comparing three models of care. *Cerebrovascular Diseases* 2007; 23: 194–202 [PubMed].

6 Rodgers H, Mackintosh J, Price C, et al. Does an early increased-intensity interdisciplinary upper limb therapy programme following acute stroke improve outcome? *Clinical Rehabilitation* 2003; 17: 579–589.

7 *Archives of Physical Medicine and Rehabilitation*, news release, Sept. 12, 2012.

8 Naqvi NH, Rudrauf D, Damasio H, Bechara A. Damage to the insula disrupts addiction to cigarette smoking. *Science* 2007; 315: 5811: 531–534.

9 House of Commons Health Committee (2005) The prevention of venous thromboembolism in hospitalised patients. London: The Stationery Office. (Guideline Ref ID: HOUSEOFCOMMONS2005).